7 Secrets of a Successful Yoga Teacher

7 Secrets of a Successful Yoga Teacher

Using the Chakras as a Guide for Teaching

DR. LISA DANA MITCHELL

This book is dedicated to my mom, who instilled in me from a young age the importance of hard work. Thanks, Mom!

Contents

Introduction

Let's be more than just *successful* as yoga teachers. Why not be *badass*? A badass yoga teacher is driven by values such as compassion, responsibility, courage, honor, humility, integrity, and selflessness. A badass yoga teacher teaches with heart and soul every opportunity he or she has to share the practice, without complaint or need for fanfare. A badass speaks the truth and lives with authenticity. A badass is someone who puts others' needs ahead of his or her own. Real badasses are often not people you likely would think are badasses, because they are humble and are in the business of serving others.

We must realize that to teach is to serve. Whether we teach Ashtanga or Iyengar, power or restorative, we all share the same mission—to help others learn to live well in their bodies, so they can live well in their lives. Although I truly believe the asanas (postures) and breath have amazing benefits to the students who practice yoga, it is the teacher who really is the icing on the cake. That icing takes a student from merely participating in a yoga class to actually *living* and *being* yoga off the mat. To be a badass yoga teacher, you have to care about two things: the student and the practice. It is easy to love the practice. But sometimes it can be hard to care for the students—they come in such a variety of levels and attitudes. There is the student who throws half a dozen questions at you the second you walk into the room. There is the student who gets up and leaves in the middle of class and never returns. The student who sighs loudly and moves quickly and impatiently, presumably because she's bored. The student who cannot connect what you are saying to his or her body and refuses to take any modifications that you offer. But still you show up, despite the feelings of fear, doubt, and loneliness this teaching profession can instill.

I wrote this book because I realize that those of us on this path of service need one another's support. We need to hold one another accountable for our actions, encourage professionalism, and embrace an ethical standard throughout the industry for our well-being and for our students' well-being. I also feel that there is so much knowledge we can take from the ancient scriptures of yoga and apply as a guide in our growth as modern yoga teachers.

In my previous book, *Don't Be an Asshole Yoga Teacher*, I use the yamas and niyamas as practical tools for teaching yoga with a high ethical standard. Now, I have employed the seven main chakras as a tool to help us understand our physical and emotional selves, deepen our connections, and be more in union with the students who show up to our classes, which will essentially make us more successful and badass yoga teachers.

First, let's have an overview of the chakra system. The word *chakra* is derived from the Sanskrit word meaning "wheel." Literally translated from Hindu culture, it means "wheel of spinning energy." A chakra is like a vortex of powerful energy. Within our bodies, we have seven of these major energy centers and many more minor ones. The seven main chakras we will focus on line the spine, starting from the base through to the crown of the head. To visualize a chakra in the body, imagine a swirling wheel of energy where matter and consciousness meet. This invisible energy, called prana, is vital life force, which keeps us vibrant, healthy, and alive.

These spinning wheels of energy correspond to massive nerve centers in the body. They regulate the flow of energy through the electrical network, or meridians, that runs through the physical body. In acupuncture and Chinese medicine, meridians are a set of pathways in the body along which vital energy is said to flow. The body's electrical system resembles the wiring in a house: it allows electrical current to be sent to every part and is ready for use when needed. Each of the seven main chakras contains bundles of nerves and major organs, as well as our psychological, emotional, and spiritual states of being. Since everything is moving, it's essential that our seven main chakras stay open, aligned, and fluid. If there is a blockage, energy cannot flow. Sometimes chakras become blocked because of stress or emotional or physical problems. If the body's energetic system cannot flow freely, it is likely that problems will occur, resulting in physical illness and/or a sense of being mentally and emotionally out of balance. Think of something as simple as your bathtub drain: if you allow too much hair to go into the drain, the bathtub will back up with water, which will stagnate, and eventually bacteria and mold will grow. This analogy can apply to our bodies and the chakras, too…though a clogged bathtub may be a bit easier to fix.

Keeping a chakra open is a bit more of a challenge, but doing so becomes easier when you have an awareness and understanding of these subtle energy centers. Since mind, body, soul, and spirit are intimately connected, awareness of an imbalance in one area will help bring the others back into balance. For example, imagine a husband who has recently lost his wife. He develops acute bronchitis, which remains in the chest, and then gets chest pains every time he coughs. The whole heart chakra is affected in this case. If he realizes the connection between the bronchitis and his being in mourning, healing will occur much faster. He would need to honor the grieving process and treat that in addition to the physical ailment.

Awareness of which of your chakras are out of balance is key to aligning them. Our bodies are in constant flux between balance and imbalance, but unless you have an apparent ailment or problem in one area of the body, imbalances can be difficult to detect. That being said, it's good to bring awareness to your body and mind and start to learn its clues as they occur. If we can build an understanding of how our own chakras, or subtle anatomy, influence the way we show up in the world as yoga teachers, it will allow us to be more able to help students find balance in their own bodies and minds.

Chakra Overview

The first three chakras, starting at the base of the spine, are more physical in nature, while the remaining four are more spiritual.

First chakra: The Muladhara is the chakra of stability, security, and our basic needs. It encompasses the first three vertebrae, the bladder, and the colon. When this chakra is open, we feel safe and fearless.

Second chakra: The Svadhisthana chakra is our creativity and sexual center. It is located above the pubic bone, below the navel, and is responsible for our pleasure and creative expression.

Third chakra: The Manipura chakra means "lustrous gem," and it's the area from the navel to the breastbone. The third chakra is our source of personal power and transformation.

Fourth chakra: Located around the area of the heart, the Anahata chakra is at the middle of the seven and unites the lower chakras of matter and the upper chakras of spirit. It is also spiritual but serves as a bridge between our body, mind, emotions, and spirit. The heart chakra is our source of love, compassion, and connection.

Fifth chakra: The Vishuddha chakra is the fifth chakra, located in the area of the throat. This is our source of verbal expression and the ability to speak our highest truth. The fifth chakra includes the neck, thyroid and parathyroid glands, jaw, mouth, and tongue.

Sixth chakra: The Ajna chakra is located between the eyebrows. It is also referred to as the "third eye" chakra. Ajna is our center of intuition. We all have a sense of intuition, but we may not listen to it or heed its warnings. Opening the sixth chakra will help your intuitive ability.

Seventh chakra: The Sahasrara chakra, also known as the "thousand-petal lotus" chakra, is located at the crown of the head. This is the chakra of enlightenment and spiritual connection to our higher selves, to others, and to the divine.

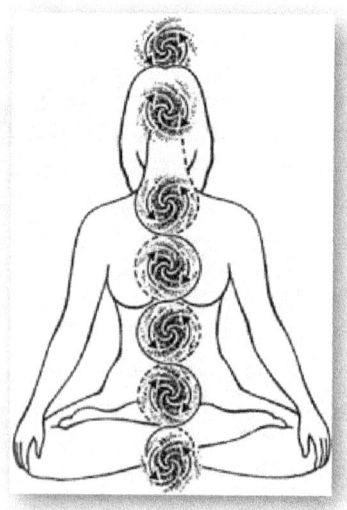

In each chapter, I have identified the key attributes and basic principles of each chakra and have provided suggestions on how to unlock a particular chakra as a yoga teacher and practitioner. I also have included some ways you can identify imbalances occurring in your life, based on characteristics of chakra excess or deficiency. I have offered a variety of suggestions that can create more energetic balance in your body and your mind as a teacher. These suggestions are based on my own journey, which I have uncovered and tested through my firsthand experience in working with countless teachers. These tools can apply directly to your teaching; they range from best practices when addressing physical bodies all the way up the chakra system to teaching yoga in a more spiritual realm. I have also included tricks to use before you teach a class, if you ever feel that a particular chakra is out of whack in your life, or if you're just not feeling as badass as you should be. As you may begin to understand, every chakra has its demon, whose intention is to hold you back from balance and being your truest self. I have offered guidance on tackling those demons, so you can show up for your students in a supportive way. Lastly, I have included a sample of poses that can complement a chakra-inspired sequence.

One

GET GROUNDED AND BE PREPARED

*To be rooted is perhaps the most important
and least recognized need of the human soul.*

—*SIMONE WEIL*

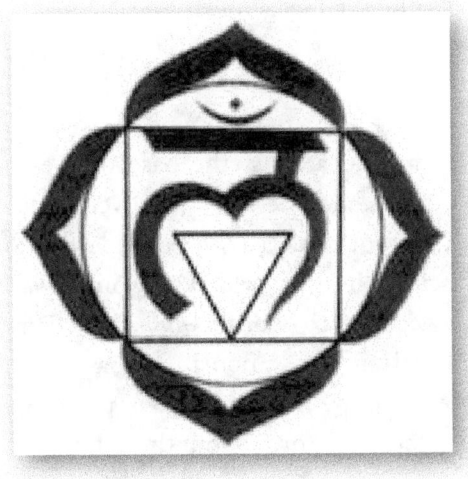

Chakra One Overview

Name: Muladhara (root)
Element: Earth
Color: Red
Purpose: Foundation
Basic Rights: The right to be here
Properties: Solid, grounded
Signs of Deficiency: Ungrounded, scattered, underweight, restless, fearful, unable to establish appropriate boundaries, anxious, showing difficulty in manifesting, resistant to structure, marked by nightmares
Signs of Excess: Lethargic, heavy, overweight, stagnant, heavy, resistant to change, marked by hoarding behaviors, subject to workaholism, prone to excessive spending
Signs of Balance: Stability, sense of safety and security, physical health, presence in the here and now, prosperity, ability to be still
Demon: Fear

Muladhara is located at the base of the spine, in the pelvic floor and the first three vertebrae around the perineum. The root chakra is responsible for your sense of safety and security in the world. The word *muladhara* breaks down into two Sanskrit words: *mula*, which means "root," and *dhara*, which means "support" or "base." As the primary basis of root support, muladhara lays the groundwork for clear energy circulation throughout the entire body. Balancing the root chakra creates the solid foundation for opening the chakras above.

Much as a building relies on the support of its foundation, a well-functioning first chakra influences clarity in all the other chakra centers. Imagine that you're laying the foundation for a house in which you're going to live for a long time (like your body). A solid foundation embedded in firm soil will provide the stability you need to create a home filled with joy and happiness for years to come. The root chakra is comprised of whatever grounds you to feel stable in your life; this includes your basic needs, such as food, water, shelter, and safety. The muladhara chakra is concerned with survival and is associated with the fight-or-flight response, so when this chakra is ignored, we are threatening our right for survival. It is critical that our foundation is strong and rooted into the ground firmly, much as roots are to a tree.

With the first chakra's relationship to survival, it is also associated with emotional needs and our ability to let go of fear. When our needs are met, we feel grounded and safe, with less overall worry from day to day. Anodea Judith, and expert on interpreting chakras in the Western world, describes quite nicely how the human body expresses its life, writing, "If your shoulders feel burdened…our body is telling us we carry too many burdens. If our knees don't want to support us, our body is telling us we don't have adequate support in our life…If our stomach has chronic pain, there is something in our life that we can't stomach…If your chest is hurting, your emotional heart is hurting." Nurturing yourself is the key to taking care of your body and keeping the first chakra happy.

When the first chakra is balanced, it signifies a belief that you have a *right to have* and the *right to be here*. The *right to be here* is closely related to the right to have. When you have a sense that you have the *right to be here*, you feel comfortable in your body, without feeling that you need to *earn* your right to exist. There is no need for justification of your needs, and you are a full participant in your life and all its decisions. Embracing *your right to have* includes having success, making time for yourself, and having friends and pleasures in life.

Whether you feel secure now often has less to do with what you have at your disposal in the present moment than it does with how safe you felt as a small child. Every chakra is related to a particular phase of growth, and the root chakra is most active between birth and seven years of age. During this early period of childhood, we are anchored to the physical world and the mother and/or father figure. We are learning safety, trust, and the innate sense of belonging (or not). When we consider psychologist Erik Erikson's stages of development, the first stage—trust versus mistrust—relates closely to the development of the root chakra. When you were an infant, if your caregivers readily and consistently gave you what you needed to survive, you felt secure in the world. You felt that the world could be trusted to provide for your basic needs. If your caregivers withheld what you needed, delayed giving it to you, or gave it to you inconsistently, you may find yourself with first-chakra blockages and imbalances. A weak muladhara chakra will damage your ability to grow as a person, to provide and nurture, and to go out into the world and fulfill your truest potential. Therefore, it's important to work with the muladhara chakra in your yoga practice to strengthen the foundations of your energy and psyche.

Often when we practice yoga, we place our attention and focus on the stability of our postures and on feeling connected and grounded to the earth beneath us. The practice is, in fact, enhancing the earth element of our being, grounding consciousness by taking our awareness from the head to the strong support systems of the legs, feet, and earth. Working on this chakra energy will make us feel calmer, stronger, and more stable. A healthy root chakra will provide a person with natural enthusiasm, confidence, motivation, and the ability to endure under stressful conditions. It produces a grounded person who feels a sense of belonging to nature and family.

Reflection:

What events or people in your past have affected your "right to be here," either positively or negatively?

What beliefs do you hold on to about these rights?

On a scale of 1–10, rate your ability to:
Remain grounded in your daily life (remain present and stay centered).

Remain grounded when someone or something is challenging you.

First Chakra Yoga-Teaching Tips

Healing for the root chakra comes from establishing a healthy connection to the body. This includes having stability within our physical surroundings and establishing healthy rituals. When considering muladhara, yoga teachers must advocate for and participate in self-care, so they can be empowered to hold space for their students. For the longest time, I thought, "What the heck does 'holding space' mean?" Well, I have discovered that *holding space* means we have to offer yoga practitioners support; we have to be available to give gentle guidance when it's needed, to offer a comfortable environment, and to let them feel safe when they make mistakes.

Get grounded. The word *grounded* can be used in many different ways: It's a verb (to ground through the feet) and an adjective (a grounded feeling). There is a certain stability associated with being grounded, for the word implies a firm footing or rootedness. When we are grounded, we are present. We are able to tap into a place of oneness with peace and equanimity, because when we find a connection to the earth, we connect to something much, much larger than ourselves. At the start of your classes, it is likely (and recommended) that you give your students a few moments to sit quietly and find some stillness as they transition into the practice. This is a powerful opportunity to allow for root-chakra establishment for the students, and I highly recommend you care for yourself in the same way. You might enjoy a few slow breaths, a few minutes of savasana, a reading of an inspirational passage, or a silent whisper of your favorite mantra before you step into the role of the teacher. This process of root-chakra integration does not take long; even five minutes can make a huge difference in minimizing your own distractions and worry. If your mind is clouded, or if you feel rushed, it will show up in your teaching. Students of yoga are intuitive beings; the unstable energy of a yoga teacher shows.

Maintain your personal practice. It's so important for yoga teachers to make physical asana a consistent practice for their own bodies. Dedication to a daily practice helps teachers to establish patience, diminish the ego, and learn how to live and teach in a more loving and supportive way. Building off the guidance above, try to avoid showing up to class without having your own opportunity for time on your mat. Remember, the root chakra is about meeting the needs of the physical, gross body. A simple practice of sun salutations, or even a simple integration of breath and movement, can be enough to get you grounded before you teach. The quality of the teacher's energy is a major factor in teaching yoga: It needs to be calm, centered, and enthusiastic. When any one of these vital ingredients is missing, your class won't be badass, regardless of the level of training and technical expertise you may have. In my opinion, the key to being grounded, calm, and attuned to the ancient practices of yoga lies in the foundation of your own personal practice.

To dig deeper with the energetics of yoga, we can integrate the *koshas*, or energy sheaths, into the discussion. The koshas are energetic layers or sheaths that move from the outermost layer of skin to the deep center of our spiritual core.

The koshas provide a framework for conceptualizing our-selves, similar to a map that explores the deepest levels of our being and can facilitate the inward journey of yoga practice. The concept of having five selves within our body appeared in the earliest yogic texts, the Upanishads. Fifteen hundred years later, Vedanta (a Hindu philosophy based on the Upanishads) refined these five selves into the koshas, the five sheaths or coverings that veil the light of our true self (known as *atman*). The koshas can be imagined as the layers of an onion, which provide a barrier that blocks us from realizing our true nature of bliss and oneness with the universe. However, yoga is a tool that enables us to peel back these layers and bring our aware-ness deeper and deeper into our bodies, eventually reaching the innermost core—our true self. When we can clearly see, harmonize, and align the layers of the koshas, we can attain a state of yoga, or oneness with the universe.

Much like the chakra system, the kosha layers come pack-aged with their own individual physiological functions and psychologies. In some respects, the kosha layers mirror the psy-chology of the chakras. The first sheath, annamaya kosha, rep-resents our physical body—our muscles, bones, ligaments, and tendons. This is the kosha most people are concerned about when they first begin a yoga practice. They generally want to tone their muscles, increase flexibility, learn to relax, gain physi-cal strength, improve balance, and find relief from the stressors of life. When you create a living connection to annamaya kosha through your own physical practice, your presence and exam-ple will be stronger for the students who show up for your class.

Lay the foundation for trust. In the modern world we live in, trust is more important than ever, especially when it comes to the relationship between student and teacher. Without trust there can be no sustainable relationship, because a relationship without trust is not really a relationship at all. It is important to acknowledge that many yoga practitioners are drawn to yoga through some hardship in their lives and either are or want to be transformed through the practice of yoga. With this in mind, honor muladhara by creating a safe environment for every person in the class. This begins from the moment a student enters the studio or practice space. Help him or her become oriented with the physical layout of the space—where the practice room is, where the restrooms and exits are located, how the mats are set up, where the props are, where the teacher will be, and so on. When you create a strong sense of security from the beginning, you can alleviate any anxiety about the class or the practice that the student may have; this is especially important for newer practitioners.

Every student deserves to feel like he or she is being cared for and protected during what sometimes can be a vulnerable space of self-exploration. This can also apply to experimenting with your flow and sequencing in your own body before you offer it to the students. If you experiment with transitions in class without practicing them yourself first, you are projecting the potential risk of the unknown onto your students. This is a violation of trust and can drain energy and confidence, both for the student and the teacher. Instead, treat your home practice as a yoga laboratory and work out the mechanics of any new poses or sequences within your own body before inviting others to do so.

Be prepared…but be flexible. Some people like to create a specific class plan, while other teachers prefer to be more spontaneous and intuitive with their teaching. Either way, a great teacher will have given time and thought to how he or she will teach a class, and that usually results in a better overall experience for the students. Preparation also takes into account arriving early, setting the scene, and creating the bhava (or vibe). There are many ways to create a desired vibe for a yoga class. Not everyone likes it, but incense is popular in Asia and can really set a tone of tranquility when the students enter. According to the Hindu tradition, the fragrant scents of incense purge the area of negative energies. An alternative to incense is burning sage. I use scents before and after class but not during; I find it can be a distraction, and smoke from incense can make breathing difficult for some students. Other ways to prepare the class vibe are to adjust the lights to fit the mood you are trying to suggest and to play music that is suitable for a yoga environment. More on music later!

Badass yoga teachers constantly adapt their teaching strategy to the students who are present. Managing such adaptation becomes second nature after years of experience, but it can be a bit more challenging to the newer teacher. I advise that you prepare classes in an intelligent way, with a specific process of safe sequencing, but be ready to throw out the prep as you see what actually presents itself in class. Why plan a flow you might not use? Because the more you work out plans and ideas when you're not teaching, the better you are able to calmly make the right choices when you *are* teaching and guiding others' practice. It is always helpful to know pose modifications and the ways props can facilitate postures. In my experience, the more advanced students know where to go. It is the beginners who will need your guidance the most. Tuning into the students' needs and being flexible with regard to a previously planned yoga flow not only demonstrates your intuition but also shows your ability to support your students. As I mentioned before, it's certainly important to plan your classes. It's great to have goals for your students, but you must also be realistic to meet the needs of that particular day and unique set of souls present in the moment. Even if you have planned the class perfectly, if your students are not ready or able to do the planned routine, what's the point?

Some days I can tell that the challenging class I have planned is exactly what the students *don't* need. They may need a more inward and relaxing class, and I am always willing to scrap any plan if I intuitively feel that doing so is necessary or would be more beneficial. Be in a place of holding space, of offering support, and you will surely see your students smiling and saying, "Thanks—that's exactly what I needed."

Establish routines. As with anything new, people are generally more at ease when they know how things work, what is going to happen, and what is required of them. One very simple way to accomplish this is to create an opening and/or closing ritual that you honor in every class. Whether it is something you say or something you do, it can give students a sense of familiarity and belonging. A routine takes away the students' feelings of anxiety by eliminating unnecessary guesswork, allowing for greater feelings of peace.

OM (or aum) is translated as a sound that encompasses all the vibrations in the universe. The sound of OM represents the beginning, the middle, and the end of all phases and cycles of life. Many yoga instructors establish the routine of beginning and ending class with the sound of OM. Chanting this mantra reminds us that we are all together in this process of practicing yoga, and it is also an effective way of drawing awareness to the vibrations within.

Namaste is a greeting that originated in the Indian subcontinent. Commonly used to mean hello or goodbye, namaste also extends to include the sentiment "I bow to the divine light in you." It is customary to bring the palms together in Anjali Mudra (hands at heart center) with a slight bow, but neither is necessary. Simply saying "namaste" includes acknowledging a pure, bright light within each of us. As with anything we say or do, the intention behind our words is what really counts.

The act of attending a yoga class alone is a ritual in itself. A ritual simply provides a sense of routine that many people crave in their lives in order to stay committed, grounded, and balanced. We are so fortunate to have the power of choice—the choice of which yoga classes to take, which teachers to study with, and which rituals we will embody in our efforts to become healthier and happier.

The Demon of Fear

When the root chakra is out of balance, there may be a manifestation of fear. This can show up as nervous energy while preparing to teach or negative self-talk during a class. Fear, however, is simply excitement with a lack of breath. If you experience fear around teaching, it is likely you are just very excited to share yoga with others, and all you may need to do to overcome the fear is breathe.

When new teachers lead their first classes, they are often overcome with fear. They worry they will make a mistake, fear they will forget their sequence, obsess that no one will show up, and so on; however, the overall consensus is that after only a few moments—often by the time they are in their second or third round of sun salutations—the fear begins to dissipate. Unfortunately, after teacher training commences, the familiar fears can quickly creep in again if you stay stagnant in your teaching opportunities. My advice for ridding yourself of any fear of teaching is simply to teach…again and again. Face your fear, so it can disappear.

Another useful strategy for overcoming fear with your teaching, as well as in other areas of your life, is to acknowledge your fear by speaking about it. When you start telling people about your fear, you take away any power it has over you. Before you speak about your fear, it exists only in your mind, and you have no way to escape from it. Get your fears out of your thoughts and into conversation with others, and you will realize there are many people who share the same concerns. This will make you feel less alone.

Another powerful tool for facing fears in your teaching is to celebrate your successes, however small they may be. In fact, I advise you to start out small: Practice teaching your friends, neighbors, and family members—whoever is willing to be your guinea pig. It is easier to face your fears of teaching strangers if you first get comfortable with a familiar support system. Every time you face your fear, celebrate your growth, and remind yourself of those successes anytime you feel afraid to move forward.

Lastly, to truly eliminate your fears around teaching, let go of your story—especially if your story sounds like this: "I am not good enough to teach yoga. I will never be good at teaching yoga. I am not good at leading groups of people, blah blah blah." Try saying those statements out loud, and you will hear how crazy they sound! These are stories your mind makes up to keep you down. Don't listen. Recognize that these are only stories. If saying your story out loud doesn't work, then try writing it down; you will quickly realize your words have no meaning unless you give it to them. Yoga teaches us that the world is our own projection; life can be a heaven or hell, based on the way we think and the stories we create. Just remember that *you* get to choose how the story goes. When you face your fear, you can connect to what you value and write a new story. Whatever the outcome of your story is, you can be an inspiration by taking action. Remind yourself that the purpose of your teaching is way more important and valuable than are any of your fears. It will pain you to not share the insightful knowledge of yoga you possess, and you'll realize you can play a part in creating a more compassionate and conscious world simply by facing your fears.

Reflection:

How much of your energy goes toward protecting yourself from fear?

What do your fears prevent you from doing that you really want to do?

What is the likelihood that your fears will truly manifest?

Before You Teach...

The root chakra regulates the sense of smell and may be soothed instantly by using grounding scents such as cedarwood, patchouli, frankincense, and clove. Before teaching class, you can apply a dab of any of these scents to your wrists or feet. Smelling these scents throughout your teaching can stabilize your breath and create more confidence and steadiness in your voice. Another way to foster feelings of security, safety, and grounding is to repeat positive affirmations such as these: *"I am safe," "The universe is a good place and is never wrong,"* and *"The universe provides for me abundantly."*

Poses to Include in a First-Chakra Sequence

1. Tadasana (mountain pose)
2. Dandasana (staff pose)
3. Supta Padangusthasana (reclined hand-to-toe pose)
4. Setu Bandha Sarvangasana (bridge pose)

5. Bhujangasana (cobra pose)
6. Adho Mukha Svanasana (downward-facing dog)
7. Utkatasana (chair pose)
8. Vrksasana (tree pose)
9. Paschimottanasana (seated forward fold)
10. Balasana (child's pose)

Two

BE FLUID AND FLOW

What do you desire?

—*ALAN WATTS*

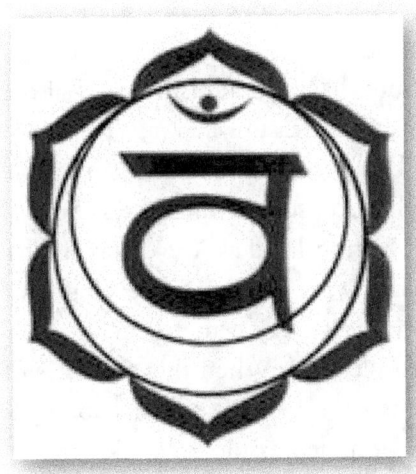

Chakra Two Overview

Name: Svadhisthana (sweetness)
Element: Water
Color: Orange
Purpose: Connection and movement
Basic Right: The right to feel
Properties: Changeable, fluid, feeling
Signs of Deficiency: Rigidity in beliefs and body, dry skin, stiff body, fear of change, avoidance of pleasure, lack of passion
Signs of Excess: Sloppy, indulgent, prone to stimulant addiction, excessively sensitive
Signs of Balance: Graceful, easy ability to embrace change, healthy boundaries, passion for life
Demon: Envy

The second chakra, svadhisthana, is also known as the creativity and pleasure chakra. This chakra is housed in the low belly between the pubic bone and navel, encompassing the genital region surrounding the sacrum. The word *svadhisthana* can be translated as "the dwelling place of the self," as it is associated with the earliest development of our identity. This feminine energy center is at the core of creativity, sensuality, and pleasure. When this chakra is out of balance, a person may experience emotional instability, fear of change, sexual dysfunction, depression, or addictions. A balanced second chakra leads to feelings of wellness, abundance, pleasure, and joy. The sacral chakra not only plays a vital role in creativity as a yoga teacher but also facilitates the development and maintenance of healthy relationships with students and peers.

In its natural state, svadhisthana brings a joyful and spontaneous expression to the self through activities such as dance, movement, exercise, and art. The nature of this chakra is to constantly seek new experiences and new challenges, because the intensity of its creative nature needs an external stimulus to fully express its potential. Through its relationship to the element of water, chakra two has a flexible, aesthetic, and inventive nature that can help us adapt to new situations. Like water, it can help us move over, under, or around life's obstacles. If this chakra energy becomes congested or blocked, we will find it harder to make positive changes to our experiences and to certain patterns of behavior, causing us to feel as though we're stuck in a cycle. Such a cycle does not bring us the love and well-being we seek or deserve, and we may be holding on—consciously or subconsciously—to the fears that prevent us from evolving into the badass people we have the potential to be.

The second chakra is concerned with our *right to feel*. A main challenge for the second chakra comes from the conditioning of our society, as we live in a society where feelings are often not valued and where passion and emotional reactions are often frowned upon. We are taught not to "lose control," causing us to disconnect from our bodies and our feelings. Culturally, this has had an enormous impact on how we deal with emotion, particularly with men, who are often made to feel that their emotions should be repressed—and women are often criticized as being weak or overly dramatic when they don't repress theirs. The suppression of feelings and emotions only serves to keep us out of touch with our emotional intelligence and sheds the *right to feel* from our experiences.

Compromise of this right can occur if you have ever been told you shouldn't feel a certain way, have been informed that your feelings were irrational or wrong, and/or if you were taught to keep your feelings to yourself. Water is the ultimate mover and changer. In order to find healing in the places we feel stuck, movement and change must occur; hence, the purpose of the second chakra is to get things moving. Without movement, there is no change, no evolution. Have you ever had an experience that you have described as really *moving*? You can see easily how connected our emotions are to this intuitive sense of movement. It is through stimulation and passion, through the fluidity and movement of the second chakra, that we can harness the power of chakra three and beyond.

Reflection:

Are you content with your life?

Do you make time for pleasure in your life?

What beliefs do you have about your emotions and ways to express your feelings?

Second Chakra Yoga-Teaching Tips

Get moving. The second chakra is related to movement, and for a yoga teacher, this means moving around the room when you teach. Long gone are the days when the yoga teacher stayed on his or her own mat at the front of the class, doing all the poses with the students. It is so difficult to feel connected to students with that outdated teaching model. You need to actually see what your students are doing in order to make suggestions on their alignment or breathing and to offer ways they can become more adept in their practice. This requires getting off your mat and moving around the room. Look at people's foundations (what body parts are on the ground). Look people in their eyes and talk them through their yoga practice. Smile. Be vulnerable. Move around so everyone can see you, but avoid moving too quickly or pacing. I highly recommend getting out of the habit of "leading" the class from the front and instead getting into the habit of "teaching" the people who show up. If you feel uncomfortable about moving around the room, the only way to overcome your discomfort is to just start doing it until it feels natural.

Many newer teachers claim to feel disoriented by getting off their mats if they were not trained to do so initially. They ponder how they will remember their flow if they aren't doing it, and they question how they'll explain the postures if they aren't embodying them. Start by coming off your mat for short sequences—remember back from chakra one: celebrate even the smallest of successes. You can build up to being off the mat for longer periods and to eventually not needing a mat of your own at all. I also recommend writing out your sequence (at least at first) so you can refer to it, if need be. That way, you are less likely to get lost or confused. As you gain confidence and experience, you will find that you need a written sequence less and less, and you will remember what order of postures you're doing more easily. There will be times you mess up or forget something; it's OK to laugh at yourself and acknowledge your mistake in a lighthearted fashion. When I first began teaching and lost my train of thought or gave a wrong cue, the phrase "I'm sorry" would immediately spill out, and I would apologize multiple times. This is a no-no: Your students have a right to feel that you're prepared and able to teach the class. If you find yourself at a loss for words or postures, practice recovering with one or more of the guidelines below:

- Take a deep breath to recenter yourself.
- Return to your notes and focus on the next posture or sequence.
- Have the yoga class take child's pose while you think through the mental lapse.
- Cue the students to take three to five deep breaths wherever they are.
- When all else fails, make a joke out of the situation and admit you're completely lost.

The second chakra is concerned with your passion and ability to have fun and be creative as a yoga teacher. You will be less confused about keeping track of your flow if you keep it simple. Start with short sequences of only two to three postures linked at a time, such as Warrior I, Warrior II, and Triangle, then transition to the other side. That way you are less likely to forget what you've done and in which order when you move on. You may need to find strategies to balance both sides equally, which can be hard when you start to give too many instructions all at once. Sometimes this can lead you to tell them everything you know about the posture on the right side, only to find you have nothing left to say on the left side. Try to start your cues from the ground up. For example, for warrior I on the right side, perhaps address the feet, legs, and hips. On the left side, build from there; address the torso, arms, and gaze. You will be giving an equal number of cues on each side and offering them something different to work on, creating a unique experience in the same pose. You can also get in the practice of counting breaths by breathing with the class, or you can use a wall clock if it has a second hand. This is a good way to make sure you don't hold your students for three minutes on the first side and ten seconds on the second side. Remember, all teachers make mistakes sometimes—even the famous ones!

Get the class moving. Do not neglect to offer Surya Namaskars (sun salutations) as a way to get fluidity and movement into your students' bodies. Sun salutations consist of a set sequence of yoga postures, traditionally done in the earlier part of a yoga practice. Sun salutations are known to enhance physical strength and prepare the body for all other postures to follow. Without a proper warm-up, the risk for yoga-related injuries increases; as a rule of thumb, sun salutations should be performed for about one-tenth of your total practice.

Energetically referring back to the koshas, as chakra one corresponded with anamaya kosha on the periphery of the body, chakra two integrates a layer deeper with pranamaya kosha. Pranamaya kosha allows more freedom in the body; the practitioner can really focus on breath exploration, particularly with the coordination of breath and body. Moving through sun salutations is a highly effective way to foster this synchronization of anamaya kosha and pranamaya kosha.

If sun salutations are done in the vinyasa style, with a linking of one breath per movement, it can provide a great cardiovascular experience. Due to the complexity of the movements and breath coordination during Surya Namaskara, concentration and focus are required. After all, the whole goal of yoga practice is to eliminate unnecessary thoughts and mind chatter. Consistent practice of sun salutation improves the functions of the heart, liver, intestine, stomach, chest, throat, and legs while purifying blood throughout the body—basically, partaking in sun salutations is a whole-body tune-up. I find that adding sun salutations to the earlier portion of a yoga class gets people connected to their bodies and their breaths while creating the internal heat of the practice. It is this heat that purifies the body, but perhaps more importantly, it purifies the mind. Neglecting to add sun salutations to your classes is neglecting the students' practices. Sun salutations not only prepare the body for all other postures to come, as I've mentioned, but I find they prepare the mind for everything else to come when we are off of our yoga mats. Pattabhi Jois (the founder of Ashtanga yoga) once said, "Practice and all is coming," but I have heard this morphed into a perhaps more pertinent phrase: "practice *because* all is coming."

Be creative in your teaching. The second chakra encourages us to be playful and exploratory as teachers. This creative energy, however, is best expressed when it builds from the stable ground of the root chakra. Therefore, before getting creative and expressive with your sequences and postures, be sure to offer stability in the body, breath, and mind. It is only then that the class can be more receptive to the unfamiliar. Never neglect an opportunity for grounding before they start to flow. Once you have established a centering and steady base, allow your creative juices to flow…but with a logic and intelligence in your sequencing.

In terms of sequencing, notice if your postures move from simple to complex. Are you allowing for both Ha and Tha (sun and moon) and sthira and sukha (strength and ease) in your sequencing? Does your sequencing support inner awareness and presence for your students? Are you creating a well-rounded yoga class that includes all the various groups of poses, with a focus on equal parts strength, flexibility, and balance? Are you moving the spine in all directions (flexion, extension, side bending, and twists)? If any of the answers to these questions are unclear, consider approaching your class structure in a different way. When you follow a basic template for a balanced yoga sequence, you can easily swap out one pose for another in the same category to keep things simple yet interesting. Below is my go-to formula, which will have students feeling a full and complete practice, but feel free to expand upon this:

- *Centering: bring the students into the space*
- *Warm-Up: gentle stretching to awaken the body*
- *Sun Salutations: these can be varied and infused, but traditional is truly perfect*
- *Standing Sequence: includes balancing postures and arm balances (optional)*
- *Backbend Sequence*
- *Core (Optional)*
- *Hip Openers*
- *Forward Folds*
- *Seated Twists*
- *Cooling Inversions, such as shoulder stand or legs up a wall*
- *Savasana*

Teaching with the intention of a peak pose to build toward can be a badass way to sequence your classes, as it introduces students to a variety of asanas while showing them an intelligent path to build upon. Once you have a pose in mind, consider what needs to be warmed up, engaged, and taught in order for your students to find some success in the apex of class, where the peak pose will be approached. Many students love the thrill of working toward a goal and value learning something specific and trying something new. Be sure to pick a pose that is appropriate to the general level of the class, especially if you are teaching a class that is considered "all levels" (a trend I find more and more studios are offering on the schedule). Here are some thoughts to consider when planning a peak-pose class:

- The pose should be challenging but not absolutely impossible.
- Make sure everyone has a stage of the final pose that is appropriate to them, so nobody feels left out.
- Take the time to really think about what your students will need to access the pose, then design a class that will enable them to cultivate whatever that is.
- Try to teach key actions and alignment principles, rather than simply shapes of poses.
- Aim to ensure you have opened the key muscle groups needed.
- Build toward the pose in a logical and progressive way.
- Make sure to leave enough time to do the appropriate counterposes in order to prepare students for savasana.

You can also teach to a particular anatomical area of the body (whether that's hips, shoulders, hamstrings, et cetera) as a way to offer creativity to a class. Teaching to a body part or region of the body is a sure way for the students to feel an activation and engagement in that particular area of the body; however, find the balance where the class still feels full and complete, touching all body parts regardless of anatomical emphasis. There truly can be so much creativity involved in class sequencing; in fact, sequencing is probably one of the reasons I love teaching Vinyasa yoga so much! With such creativity, however, there is much room for error. If you strive for balance in a class, you likely will make your students happy. Balance in a yoga class is an art and will become stronger the more you teach and hone your craft. Some simple guidelines that can help you find this balance are listed below:

- Be sure you are spending just as much time strengthening the backside of the body as you spend on the front.
- Take the time to stretch the quads, chest, shoulders, and hip flexors, as these areas are often overused and under stretched.
- Spend intentional time in grounded and seated postures, as these often mirror standing poses and aid in the class cool down.
- Facilitate humble, quiet introspection. This balances out the on-the-go energy that exists in the business of life off the mat.
- Don't cheat their savasana; some yogis consider this to be the most important posture of all, as savasana allows the body to heal and has many meditative

qualities. Hold and honor this important space for your students.

In terms of creativity, keep in mind that new teachers often feel pressured to constantly change their sequences. More experienced teachers stay creative but focus on keeping aspects of class more consistent for students. From my experience, most students prefer a certain amount of routine with just enough variations to keep things feeling fresh and alive when they practice. I often recommend that during a new teacher's first year of teaching, he or she should make only minimal changes to the flow, if any.

Be changeable. The second chakra's element is water, and the greatest teaching that comes from water is adaptability. In its fluid form, water does not resist obstacles. Without effort, it simply adjusts its form, shape, and direction to adapt to its surroundings. As Bruce Lee said, "Be like water." Be willing to leave out aspects of your planned sequence if you realize it may be too challenging for your group, or be ready to add in more advanced postures if most of them seem up for it.

As a teacher, you must be ready for anything to happen. You'll experience everything from weird noises emitting from people's bodies and private parts hanging out of clothing to overflowing toilet water running into the studio and practitioners arguing in the middle of class. These are all things I have experienced as a yoga teacher, so be fluid, flexible, and ready for anything! That's badass.

Learn people's names. This is good advice for everyone, but it is particularly important for those who have opened themselves up to being teachers. People love to hear their names; when we feel acknowledged and known, we feel valued. Research suggests that when a teacher knows the names of his or her students, it improves the overall climate of the class or studio atmosphere. People also love when you ask and remember interesting details of their lives. I am not suggesting you stalk each student on social media until you know their entire life by heart—that would be creepy—but do ask how their day was, what they do for a living, their vacation plans, and so on. Once you have gathered all this information, expand upon it and continue to bring it up in conversation. It not only shows that you care but also makes the student feel loved and important.

Maintain healthy boundaries with the students who come to your classes. In the event that you become more than first-name-basis friendly with the practitioners who come to your class—meaning you gather socially outside of the studio—you must be clear about the distinction between the student-teacher relationship and other relationships that have developed. You must also be wary of relationships that create energetic imbalance. You must consider that when you are a yoga teacher, you are holding a safe space for a student to learn and grow on the path of yoga. When you enter into a more personal relationship with that student, boundaries can become blurred quickly.

For example, if you spent an hour with your therapist describing in-depth details of an issue from your past, then met him or her later that night for drinks, it could create enormous confusion for both parties. You may not even feel safe going back to that therapist, as now the value of what he or she offers has been diminished through a casual exchange. I have personally struggled with this, because I encounter so many amazing individuals through the studios and our teacher-training programs. Yet due to my own experience with lines becoming blurred through friendship, I no longer look at students in my classes or training programs as the individuals to appease my social needs. I am also mindful of what details I share with them about my personal life. It's only once a student becomes a peer and stops seeking me out as a mentor that I enter into a more personal friendship.

In terms of intimate sexual relationships with students, I suggest steering clear. In any other teaching profession, if teachers have sexual relations with students, they may be stripped of their certificate or license and are removed from their role. Yet in the business of yoga, sexual transgressions with students seem to happen far too often. If you truly believe the love of your life has entered the studio and is learning yoga from you, I suggest you advise him or her to stop taking your classes, so you are no longer his or her teacher. Enough said.

Teach with joy. If you're not having fun or radiating joy when teaching, then yoga is becoming just another chore for you. When teachers experience "yoga teacher burnout," I wonder whether the inner joy of their personal practice has also disappeared. Without a personal practice, your teaching enthusiasm won't last long. So many teachers struggle with finding the balance between teaching and practicing, and there have been times in my own teaching career that I have felt my personal practice was slipping away. Here are a few guidelines to call upon if you are struggling with your personal practice:

- Find a teacher whose classes and teaching style resonate with you. Go to his or her classes as often as you can.
- Just get on the mat. Some days you may practice for an hour; other days you may practice for fifteen minutes. Both types of practices have benefits, so don't feel badly about a shorter practice. Instead, be grateful you had time on your mat. I have a friend who will drink her coffee on her yoga mat, as she truly believes that being on the mat, in any capacity, helps.
- Establish a routine. Create a time of day that you practice, and keep it consistent.
- Sometimes you can't make it to a class. Have a home practice. When you have a home practice, have a designated space for it. Have your mat and any props in place so you don't waste any time with setup. (This may require you to set up the night before if you are an early-morning practitioner.)

Yoga teachers, we are not just sharing information on yoga alignment. We are sharing information on a way of being. Maintain your practice, as it is through practice that you can continue to teach with joy and enthusiasm. Commit to your practice. Again, this devoted practice need not consume hours of your day, but it should leave you feeling nourished and revived when you teach.

The Demon of Envy

One of the primary emotional symptoms of second-chakra imbalance is envy. This demon is something to be aware of in yourself and in your students. The easiest way to alleviate the potential for jealousy is to celebrate success and desirable qualities in others. In doing so, we acknowledge these attributes as a reflection of the best parts of ourselves. In Yoga Sutra 1.33, Patanjali encourages us to "delight in the virtuous," meaning we should admire those who embody qualities we wish to have and follow their example, rather than harboring feelings of envy and insecurity. I admit—in this generation of Instagram yoga stars, with their slim bodies and graceful yoga transitions—it is difficult to not have feelings of envy and inferiority. I think many yoga teachers can understand this confession, and I know many who need breaks from social media just to clear their heads of negative and envious thoughts. Instead of harboring feelings of envy toward teachers who have better-attended classes, remind yourself that you can't be the best teacher for everyone, and that's OK.

On the other hand, adding a bit of friendly competition into the practice has been helpful for me and has even made me more consistent and invested in my personal practice. But I have changed the way I think about yoga over the years. I know asana is only one-eighth of this beautiful eight-limbed path, so now I think, "I will use my ujjayi breath better than you…I will fall out of handstand better than you…I will relax in savasana better than you." Reminding myself of this keeps me consistent, and I can see more clearly that I don't need ten more years of practice to finally get a handstand into a crow pose and don't need to lose twenty more pounds to get both legs behind my head easily. I am content with my practice as it is, in each and every changing moment and in each and every changing breath. What a great concept to remind students of again and again until it sinks in.

Reflection:

Where do you resist movement and change in your life (e.g., moving toward new relationships, jobs, or experiences)?

Before You Teach…

Eating or drinking orange or sensual foods is a fast way to enhance your second chakra before you teach. Oranges and mangos are two excellent choices. A piece of dark chocolate will do the trick, too. These indulgent treats stimulate the pleasure centers in the brain and immediately put you into second-chakra zone.

Poses to Include in a Second-Chakra Sequence:

1. Supta Baddha Konasana (reclined bound-angle pose)
2. Ananda Balasana (happy baby pose)
3. Baddha Konasana (bound-angle pose)
4. Upavistha Konasana (seated wide-legged forward fold)
5. Uttan Pristhasana (lizard pose)
6. Eka Pada Kapotasana (king pigeon pose)
7. Agnistambhasana (fire log or double pigeon pose)

Three

BUILD CONFIDENCE AND AUTHENTICITY

That which does not kill us makes us stronger.

—*FRIEDRICH NIETZSCHE AND KANYE WEST*

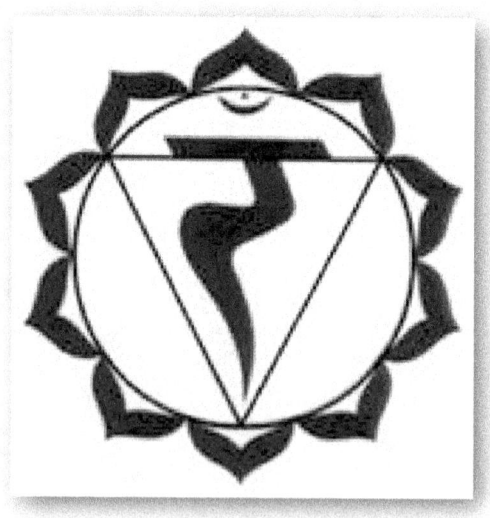

Chakra Three Overview

Name: Manipura (lustrous gem)
Element: Fire
Color: Yellow
Purpose: Transformation
Basic Rights: The right to act, to be a unique individual
Properties: Strength, heat, power, energy
Signs of Deficiency: Weak will, low energy, low self-esteem, passive, attraction to stimulants
Signs of Excess: Overly aggressive, controlling and manipulative in relationships, prone to sedatives abuse, frequent temper tantrums, competitive nature, hyperactive
Signs of Balance: Reliable, good self-esteem, confident, responsible, able to face challenges, sense of humor, balanced ego
Demon: Shame

The journey of the chakra begins with earth, moves to water, and then flows to fire. When you feel grounded and your emotions are flowing, you can create some transformative energy. The third chakra, manipura, is often called the power chakra. Manipura is located around the navel in the area of the solar plexus. It is a masculine source of personal radiance and power that governs self-esteem, energy, and the ability to manifest and transform.

An excessive third chakra can elicit aggression and ego-driven behavior, and when the third chakra is deficient, it will deplete energy and foster low self-esteem. It is sometimes easier to identify the symptoms of a chakra when it is unbalanced, because symptoms go to polar extremes and are more clearly defined. If manipura becomes exacerbated, symptoms may show as excessive heat in the body, high blood pressure, hot flashes, and sweating. Our personality may become more aggressive and domineering, and we may seek power over others and try to control a situation where we feel we are losing control. Fortunately, the third chakra has the power to recognize its own shortcomings and the strength to change quickly and harness its fiery drives in support of the whole. If stress causes manipura to become underactive instead of overactive, the opposite symptoms will occur: lack of body heat, low blood pressure, feeling cold all the time, apathy, lacking in self-esteem, and the inability to commit to the completion of projects and/or obligations.

When manipura is strong and healthy, its natural fire will radiate confidence, warmth, well-being, and friendliness. Because manipura is related to light, fire, and sight, the mind becomes clearer, and thoughts and actions become organized. A balanced third chakra allows control of ourselves and our lives, making us better able to make decisions quickly and extract essential meanings from the situations going on around us. Individuals with a healthy third chakra present as warm-hearted, natural leaders or positive centers of influence.

The life lesson given to this chakra pertains to handling power for the betterment of humanity. It requires strength and vision to handle power correctly, and fortunately, manipura is blessed with both of these qualities; however, power can easily be abused, making traits that are manipulative, pushy, and persuasive, often hidden under the false pretense of altruistic causes. We can see this awful trait in some politicians, who are driven by ambition and vanity and who will say almost anything to obtain influence and power.

The basic right of the third chakra is the *right to act*. It is through action that we find the strength to move forward and make changes and transformations to ourselves and the world around us. As fire transforms to heat, the third chakra governs our digestion and metabolism, so awareness of your food intake and how what you eat corresponds to your energy level are key components to finding balance within this chakra. As yoga teachers, every time we step into a studio, we rely on manipura to navigate the teaching role with confidence and grace. Having a strong internal fire is what gives us the spark to make change and transformation in our lives. In yoga, we call this fire *tapas*, or discipline. Tapas is a combination of personal will, concentration, and practice, and it is through these applications that we can burn the blockages in our lives that hold us back from revealing and being our true selves. Interestingly enough, humans are the only animals able to have a sense of control over fire. We are also the only animals capable of complex acts of will. As yoga teachers and practitioners, it is important that we harness the immense power we are capable of to transform our positive intentions into reality. By living with intention, discipline, and will, we have the responsibility to create a life on purpose.

Chakra three is also the center of the trinity of matter, energy, and consciousness. In the spiritual texts of yoga, we refer to this as the three *gunas,* or qualities of nature: *tamas, rajas,* and *sattva.* All three gunas are always present in all beings and objects surrounding us, but the qualities that dominate will vary and fluctuate, though the predominant guna acts as a lens that affects our perceptions and perspective of the world. Unlike other objects or animals, humans have the unique ability to consciously alter the levels of the gunas in our bodies and minds through practices of yoga, the quality of our thoughts, and the lifestyle practices we choose.

Without even realizing it, you've probably occasionally felt tamasic, just wanting to lie around and binge watch a show. Other days, you have a ton of energy (rajasic), take two yoga classes in a day, and clean your whole house from top to bottom. Yet other days, you may feel remarkably calm and insightful (sattvic)—maybe like your favorite yoga teacher. This means that our transient moods and permanent personalities can generally be characterized according to the gunas. Here is a further explanation of the qualities that represent the three gunas.

Tamas is a state of darkness, inertia, inactivity, and materiality. Tamas manifests from ignorance and deludes all beings from their spiritual truths. To reduce tamas, avoid oversleeping, overeating, inactivity, passivity, and fearful situations. Tamasic foods include heavy meats and foods that are spoiled, chemically treated, processed, or refined.

Rajas is a state of energy, change, and movement. The nature of rajas is of desire and attachment. Hence, rajas binds us to the fruits of our labor and can be a cause of suffering. To reduce rajas, avoid overexercising, overworking, loud music, excessive thinking, and overconsumption and desire of material goods. Rajasic foods include fried foods, spicy foods, and caffeine.

Sattva is a state of balance, joy, and intelligence. Sattva is often referred to as the state of the yogi, as it reduces rajas and tamas, making liberation possible. The yogic practices were developed to create sattva in the mind and body; therefore, practicing yoga and leading a yogic lifestyle strongly cultivates this peaceful nature. To increase sattva, reduce both rajas and tamas by enjoying activities that produce joy and positive thoughts. Sattvic foods include whole grains, legumes, and fresh fruits and vegetables that grow above the ground.

As a badass yoga teacher, it is useful to find a balance between all three gunas in your classes. Strive to simultaneously guide students to be grounded to the earth (tamas); passionate about yoga (rajas); and reaching for the ultimate goal, which is the realization of the authentic self (sattva).

Reflections:

What naturally increases your energy? What drains it?

Do you utilize your energy wisely by keeping realistic goals?

Third Chakra Yoga–Teaching Tips

Be confident in your teaching. Studies indicate that people with healthy self-confidence are generally happier and more satisfied with their lives than are people who lack self-confidence. Confidence can help you approach the world with more energy, enthusiasm, and determination, resulting in better relationships, higher-quality work, and a feeling of being connected with your surroundings. Self-confident people are more able to influence others and control their own emotions and behaviors more responsibly. A positive attitude results from feeling good about yourself and knowing your place in the world is important and meaningful. People who embrace strong levels of confidence are more relaxed in social settings and when engaging with new people. Because their belief in themselves is internal and not reliant on the judgment of others, they can move about freely, without fear of rejection. Confident people tend to attract people to them, as such positive energy is contagious and appealing.

Teaching yoga is a sacred responsibility, yet it is natural for a new teacher to feel nervous and question his or her ability to lead a class. It's important to remind yourself that regardless of how many classes you have under your belt, the students in the class are still depending on you for guidance and support. Step confidently into this role and be secure in knowing you are up to the task—you do have what it takes. Speak firmly and with conviction, and do not hesitate to give instructions. Exemplify your passion for yoga, and your confidence in your students becomes a reflection of your own confidence and enthusiasm concerning the practice.

This will occasionally mean you have to take a stand for a student's safety (telling him or her to modify a pose to avoid injury, for example) or have a difficult conversation with a student, but this is the important work of the third chakra. You may recall an insecure internal dialogue from when you were a newer yoga student, as it is more common than not for new practitioners to take physical adjustments and modifications from the teacher as an insult. It's easy to assume you're being adjusted because you're wrong. It's important to remind students that we all start off doing poses without the poses' optimal benefits, whether these are focused on alignment, focus, or how one integrates breath. It is impossible to walk into your first class and be accurate on every minute detail; however, it is our job to identify students who could potentially harm themselves and to prevent injury. Any adjustments made or specific guidance should not be driven by ego, but rather should come from the desire for the student to grow and understand the postures on a deeper level. Every time you offer an adjustment to a student, it should come from a place of concern, nurturance, and support.

Let go of the ego. The amazing thing about the universal teachings in Patanjali's Yoga Sutras is that the 196 threads (sutras) pertain primarily to the mind. The collection discusses in great detail the qualities of the mind and the ways we can eliminate incorrect thought, referred to as *kleshas*, or clouding of the mind. One main facet of the Yoga Sutras is the discussion on our perceptions. If we can witness how we perceive situations, we can then learn how we often create our own problems. Even better, the Yoga Sutras suggest we can free ourselves of our problems, if only we can better understand our perceptions. The Yoga Sutras define two terms, *avidya* and *vidya*. *Avidya* translates to "incorrect comprehension," or false perceptions. The opposite, is *vidya*, which translates to "correct understanding." *Avidya* becomes engrained in our way of being, due to habits we become dependent on, as well as unconscious actions that accumulate over time. These habits and accumulations are our *samskaras,* or imprints, which cover our minds with incorrect understanding. The goal of yoga is to peel away the branches of avidya, so we can notice when our perceptions are wrong, essentially giving the practitioner a clear lens through which to understand and view their actions, the actions of others, and the world around them.

One important factor to consider with avidya is that these instances of ignorance are sneaky and hide well from our understanding; however, I will shed some light on the four main causes of our suffering, as defined by Patanjali's Yoga Sutras:

- Asmita a.k.a. the ego: The ego creates the idea that we must be better than someone else, and/or we must always be right. I see this often yoga classes when practitioners are comparing themselves to others or are pushing themselves too hard, as if to prove a point. This element of ego can create feelings of inferiority, when the practice of yoga is intended to make us feel content and calm.
- Raga: This is the branch of avidya that makes us want something today because it was pleasant yesterday or even makes us just imagine that something may be

wonderful, creating a sense of desire. Overall, it is the sense that we want things we don't have, even when those things aren't good for us. It is the feeling that what we have is not enough—a sense of overall dissatisfaction about our blessings. Raga can also be evident in our not wanting to let go of what we already have.

- Dvesa: In many ways, dvesa is the opposite of raga. It is a sense of rejection. This might entail rejecting things with which we are not familiar or the inability to step out of our comfort zones. Dvesa also becomes apparent when we are afraid of an experience because it once brought us pain (e.g., maybe your heart was once broken, and now you are afraid to love again).
- Abhinivesa: Fear. Often abhinivesa is the most secretive of all the branches of avidya. It involves our feelings of doubt and uncertainty.

It is through these four clouds of the mind that we find dissatisfaction and suffering in our lives. If we can recognize when avidya is affecting our state of mind, we can make sound judgments in our life choices. We can tell when we are seeing things correctly, because we can notice peacefulness inside of us. Only when avidya is in action do we feel tension and agitation. Take some time to notice avidya when it creeps in; become a witness to your mind. The wonderful thing about yoga is that it makes avidya more apparent. With a consistent yoga practice, you may even notice more vidya, or correct understanding, coming to surface.

In terms of ego, there are a few key ways to identify whether your ego is taking over your life: Do you always need to be right? When others offer constructive criticism or question your actions, do you politely disregard their input and continue to do things the way you've always done them? After all, you should know best, right? The yoga world can be so competitive, despite all the teachings that preach contentment, avoidance of judgment, and peace within yourself. As a yoga teacher, are you in constant competition with someone who probably doesn't think much about you at all? This could be anyone, from the latest Instagram yoga sensation to an old lover or former college roommate. If you spend more time and energy than you care to admit (even to yourself) devising a way to outdo this person or prove to the world that you are more successful, you may have a problem with your ego.

Do you seek constant approval and others' recognition? True, we all desire approval and recognition to a certain degree, but do you thrive on the favorable opinion of others (rather than the peace that comes from knowing you are following a divine plan)? Are you barely satisfied or content with your accomplishments? Each time you reach a new level of success or achieve a goal, do you make a mental list of all the ways you could have done it differently (or better!) and then quickly set your sights on the next big dream? It takes a tremendous amount of honesty and humility to admit you identify with any of these signs of inflated ego. But I want you to know that when I was guilty of these behaviors (and I've been guilty of them all at one point or another), it was very clear to everyone except me.

Since the ego is the ultimate expression of power, confidence, and will, it is easily prone to manipura-related imbalance. Despite its eagerness to show itself, the ego has no place in a yoga practice. Let this be your mantra— Teaching yoga is about being of service to others, it has nothing to do with me. The yogic scriptures teach us that we are not this moment, we are not this thought, and we are not this pain or this suffering. Therefore, we should also remind ourselves as teachers that we are not amazing, we are not the best, and we are not the worst. A yoga teacher is simply sharing the practice. A badass teacher doesn't make it about them; they make it about the practice of yoga and all the many benefits we gain when yoga is practiced consistently and without interruption.

A great learning tool is to request questions or feedback after you teach a class. Try not to let your ego become inflated when your students praise you and your teaching style, and at the same time, do not get your feelings hurt if your class attendance is low. It takes only one student to make you a teacher, and there are many reasons students can't show up to practice. Life just gets in the way sometimes, or maybe the universe just has other plans for them that day. Teaching yoga is such a fulfilling and incredible job, and it is a job that comes with both criticism and accolades. For the most part, accolades are the dominant of the two forms of feedback, and learning to not attach yourself too strongly to positive feedback is an important part of taming your ego and keeping the third chakra in a state of balance.

Have a sense of humor. Laughing has been shown to improve your immune system by helping the body produce more infection-fighting materials while lowering the amount of stress hormones in the body. In addition, laughing has been shown to relax one's muscles and lowers blood pressure, making it a great way to reduce chances of heart attack or stroke. More obviously, laughing improves your mood and helps you feel better about yourself and life in general. In fact, there is even a style of yoga, called Laughter yoga, that promotes the use of laughter as a form of physical exercise. Laughter yoga was created in India in the mid-1990s and has quickly grown as a grassroots social movement of independent community laughter clubs, promoting the ideal of a nonpolitical, nonreligious, nonracial, nonthreatening, and noncompetitive simulated approach to laughter. Its core premise is that your body can and knows how to laugh, regardless of what your mind has to say. Because it follows a body-mind approach to laughter, participants do not need to have a sense of humor, know jokes, or even be happy. The premise is to "laugh for no reason," faking laughter until it becomes real.

When manipura is balanced, we are able to experience enthusiasm and joy in our teaching. Humor can loosen up the atmosphere in a class, as laughter and lightness tend to make people feel more comfortable and relaxed. Adding a bit of comedic relief in a yoga class can remind us we are all human, and any nervous energy can dissipate through laughter. Seeing someone smile is encouraging and joyful. It's always fun to see people smile, and since humor depends on surprise, it creates a true sense of being present. Also, a teacher should use each talent he or she has in teaching. Use your entire personality as a teacher; be vulnerable and present, and if you have the capability to be humorous, why shouldn't you be?

Empower students. Most of the classes I teach are considered all-levels classes, meaning there are people in the class who are brand new to yoga, mixed in with students who have been practicing for many years. Your classes will likely have this variance at times, too. Therefore, I suggest you emphasize to the students that their practices are their own. Encourage them to realize that each of their experiences is unique, and that they are their own most important teacher. This gives students the ability to take the practice into their own hands, rather than always relying on a teacher to tell them what to do. It can also have ramifications for living their yoga off the mat, helping the student to realize he or she has the power and ability to make choices for himself or herself, in all areas of life. You can create a culture of empowerment with your students by using key phrases in your teaching dialogue. Some phrases I recommend are listed here, but feel free to find the words of power and encouragement that work for you.

- *Trust your intuition.*
- *You are your own best teacher.*
- *Find the variation that feels good to you.*
- *Comparison is the thief of joy.*

- *Your yoga mat is your own private island.*
- *Let go of the concern of what other people are doing around you.*
- *If it doesn't feel good, please come out of the pose.*

A core element of reducing the imbalance of the power relationship between yoga teacher and student can start with the belief that the student is the expert of their own body—and life, for that matter. With any teacher-student relationship, there is an uneven power dynamic that cannot be denied or completely erased, but with awareness and consciousness of the subject, we can minimize this imbalance. There is a fine line between sharing knowledge and presenting as the authority, but the differentiating factor is the attitude the teacher displays. Be an instrument of empowerment when you teach.

Offer props. By openly stating that there are many variations based on each individual body and experience level, you can encourage students to accept their variations matter-of-factly, recognizing that they are not flawed but simply learning their own customized way of expressing the pose. It is important to teach students to recognize what each asana looks like, regardless of the countless ways individual bodies may take the pose. B. K. S. Iyengar introduced props into the modern practice of yoga to allow all practitioners access to the postures' benefits, regardless of age, physical condition, or experience level. The central purpose for using yoga props is to address a need for support. A "prop" is just that: it is supportive and helpful when facing obstacles on the mat, because it helps the practice to meet the student where he or she is. In all my years of teaching, I have yet to find one person who didn't benefit from using a yoga prop in one way or another in a yoga class. I try to encourage the students in the belief that props are not simply for beginners but can be a tool to enhance the practice in a multitude of ways. From the strongest, most flexible practitioner to the brand-new beginner, a strategically placed yoga prop can elevate the physical and spiritual trajectory of yoga practice.

There have been countless times that I have taken the initiative to get blocks for a student who was struggling to touch the floor. Even after I put the blocks right next to the student's hands, he or she sometimes ignores them and continues to struggle. All the struggling does is reinforce bad habits, because somehow he or she is convinced that using a prop is a bad thing. Perhaps the beginner believes it's not cool or makes them a less-than or even bad yogi if they use a prop here and there. What they don't realize is that those people kicking up into advanced inversions and arm balances most certainly used some type of support along the way in order to get to where they are now. Therefore, I advise you to offer props for all your students before the class begins. That way no one feels less-than, and in the event that you offer a block under someone's hand in half-moon pose, it feels more like being guided than like being punished, as the block is readily available and suggested for all. Hold the space for students to honor their bodies by using props to allow the practice to meet them exactly where they are and as they are.

The yoga block is the most versatile and frequently used prop found in the yoga room. The block is designed with three different heights and is used to assist with alignment and to provide extra reach when muscles feel tight. Blocks are highly effective in a variety of poses and transitions. Here are a few common block opportunities:

- Forward fold: To loosen tight hamstrings, have students separate their feet hips-width distance apart with a block under each hand. They can bend their knees slightly and fold forward by hinging at their hips. With the support of their blocks, they can relax their torso (especially the head and neck) down toward the floor.

- Triangle: If students are having a hard time lengthening their torsos while reaching toward the floor, place a block on the floor on the inside of the front foot. This may be more appropriate than having them place their hand on their shin, big toe, or mat.

- Half-moon: Cue the students to place the block about one foot in front of the toes of their balancing leg. This extra height and support will help students focus on stacking their shoulders and hips, making the floor more accessible and allowing the standing leg to be a straight, solid base.

- Half pigeon: In half pigeon, it's important for students to keep their hips square and aligned with the front edge of their mat. If you see a struggle with this alignment, place a block under their right buttock when their right leg is forward in half pigeon, then under the left buttock when their left leg is forward.

- Supported bridge: Sometimes we all need a little extra support. Have the students come to bridge pose and place the block under their sacrum, the flat part of their back at the base of their spine. The height of the block depends on the student's back flexibility.

Yoga straps are useful to achieve poses that address tight shoulders and/or hamstrings, but teachers can definitely get creative with their uses:

- Seated forward fold: When students are in a seated position with their legs extended forward, instruct them to wrap the strap around their feet and hold one end in each hand. Prompt them to move their hands up the strap closer to their feet, coming deeper into the forward fold. This modification is for yogis who struggle with tight hamstrings and can't reach their ankles or feet in a seated forward fold.
- Reclined hamstring stretch: Students can lie on their back and loop the strap around one foot. With the leg extended straight up toward the ceiling, they can hold on to the strap with both hands, pulling their leg toward their body, head toward the knee.
- Gomukhasana (cow-face pose): Are you noticing students having a hard time clasping their hands in

cow-face pose? They can hold one end of the strap in their right hand with their arms straight up in the air. Then, cue them to bend their right elbow, so their hand dangles between their shoulder blades. With a bend of their left elbow behind them, they can grab the strap and inch their left hand toward their right hand, and vice versa.

- Forward fold with hands clasped: This popular forward-fold variation is difficult for yogis with tight shoulders. Instead of interlacing their hands at their lower back, they can separate them slightly by using the strap. Prompt them to fold forward and let their hands move toward the ceiling. They may need to loosen their grip on the strap and move their hands farther apart to ease into the shoulder stretch.

- Standing side bend with arms overhead: Have them hold their strap with their hands one or two feet apart and their arms reaching overhead. Instruct them to bend to the right, then to the left, a few times.

The bolster is typically utilized for reclined, restorative, or seated poses. It provides a little lift off the floor and a cushion that eases the body into relaxation. Offer these bolster variations to common yoga postures:

- Elevated legs up a wall: When students place their legs up the wall per usual, have them lift their hips. Slide a bolster underneath.

- Reclined heart opener: From a seated posture with legs extended forward, students can lie back with the bolster starting at their lower back and stretching up to their head. Try this pose in place of fish or other heart openers.
- Bolster under knees for savasana: cue them to come to corpse pose with a bolster under their knees.
- Supported child's pose: Have students kneel and pull the bolster between their legs. They can lie facedown, resting the front of the body on the bolster.
- Reclined hero's pose: students can come to a seated hero's pose and lie back to rest their spine and head on the bolster.

The yoga blanket, similar to the bolster, is great for extra padding or a boost of height. Keep a blanket nearby for the following pose variations:

- Shoulder stand: Have students pad their shoulders and upper back with the blanket. This can help to keep the natural curve in the cervical spine in the shoulder-stand position.
- Headstand: if a student is new to headstand or looking to stay there for a long time, a folded blanket can provide a softer base.
- Easy seated pose: When staying in seated pose for an extended period of time, yogis should situate their hips higher than their knees. This can be achieved by

using a block, bolster, or blanket (the tighter the hips, the more height you'll need).

- Under the knees for padding: If students prefer extra padding under their knees in tabletop or other poses, have them keep a blanket next to their mat for additional support, as needed.
- Covering in savasana: Use the blanket as, well, a blanket! During savasana, students can use it to cover their bodies as they rest and relax.

Tune in to your motivation for music. There's a widespread debate in the yoga world over the efficacy and relevance of music in a yoga class, so it's important to ask yourself what your motivation is for the music you choose. *Why* you play a piece of music in class is just as, if not more, important as what you play. I feel it is important to discuss music for the third chakra, as it has a relationship to exerting a sense of power in the classroom. Classes without music can also be highly meditative, as the silence teaches self-observation and acceptance of what is going on in our bodies and in the chatter of our minds.

It brings to mind a class I took at a local studio recently. It happened to be the day after the Country Music Awards were on, and the teacher started the class by saying, "I hope you all like country music, because that's my entire playlist today!" Needless to say, I am not a fan of country music, but I used that opportunity to really practice some yoga, tuning out the sounds that were inherently distracting for me and forcing myself to go more inward. Although I am sure the teacher had no ill intentions in having a playlist of only one genre of music, a genre she clearly preferred, her decision was not essentially in line with putting students first or in a place of empowerment. We clearly had no choice but to listen to country songs for an hour.

I generally am a fan of music when I practice and teach, but I do believe in some guidelines. First, let's talk about some of the cons of playing music while you teach. Often, newer teachers use music as an indulgence, or a way to seek a diversion to hide their own insecurities. You may also feel that music helps to entertain or fill gaps of silence or awkwardness, but often those gaps of silence and awkwardness are exactly where the magic can happen for the students. Silence itself has a sound. Without music, there can still be song through the breath (perhaps the greatest soundtrack of all), the beating of your heart, or the sounds of nature that may be happening right outside the studio. Be mindful that music can hide the subtleties of the beauty happening inside of the individual.

You must also keep in mind the ear of the beholder. As I mentioned, people's musical taste are different, and not everyone in the class will have the same musical preferences. In addition, music can be highly personal. You can play a song that takes a person back to a specific situation or time of life and elicit past memories (good or bad); a song can quickly take them out of the present moment of the practice. Consider the volume you are using, as well, as that can be a distraction. Generally, any volume over one hundred decibels is uncomfortable for people, and it can result in students straining to hear the teacher's cues over the music. On the other hand, music that is too soft can have the students feeling like the music is just a tease. Again, music that is not planned and executed mindfully can be just another distraction from the flow of the class and the changes students can experience.

But does playing music in yoga class prevent us from finding stillness, or can it help us to deepen the practice? This is definitely based on the individual, so I always tell teachers in my teacher-training program that you will never please everyone, especially when it comes to music. Dopamine is released in the brain when we listen to music, and that's a feel-good chemical essential for the functioning of the central nervous system. So there is no doubt that music can be very soothing for the soul. Music can definitely make a class unique, especially when the music is planned to correspond to what is happening in the class. Just as a class starts off mindful, grounding, and slower paced to awaken the body, the music should start that way, too. When the class gets moving, say through sun salutations and standing poses, the music should represent more vigor and excitement to inform and correspond to the energy of the class. As the class cools down, slows down, or begins the descent to savasana, the music should be indicative of that, too. Definitely be specific about the song you play for savasana; it must be calm and soothing to not take away from students' experience in this critical part of the class. If you are unsure, let there be silence in savasana.

As for pop music, I stand by the 80 percent rule. In a seventy-five-minute class, I would recommend not exceeding three or four (twelve minutes or so) of songs you may recognize from the radio. There really is no right or wrong where music is concerned; it all depends on different tastes and different moments in your life. The most important thing is that people are practicing yoga, whether it's to MC Yogi or to the sound of their breath.

The Demon of Shame

When the third chakra is imbalanced, shame is often one of the most common emotional indicators. According to the *Merriam-Webster* dictionary, shame is defined as a feeling of guilt, regret, or sadness that you have because you know you have done something wrong. Shame is a self-conscious emotion and brings upon feelings of inadequacy, unworthiness, dishonor, or regret. Shame can be triggered by another person, circumstances, or by your own perceived failures. Given that shame can lead you to feel as though your whole self is flawed, bad, or subject to exclusion, it makes you want to withdraw or hide your true self.

As a teacher, you may experience shame, particularly as it relates to any aspect of your teaching. Therefore, I beg you to be kind to yourself in your thoughts, words, and actions. Do not allow yourself to dwell on any particular part of class that you perceive as subpar or question if you should have done things differently. It is so easy to shame ourselves, when chances are students do even notice the same intricacies we do about ourselves and our teaching. Forgive yourself when you forget something in your sequence, mess up right and left, or mince your words. Your students will forgive you, so you should, too. The negative mind chatter can go on and on, unless you have it in your awareness and stop it. Those moments of awareness and introspection can bring us the most profound growth, and those opportunities help us shape our teaching for the next time we are given the opportunity.

If you make a mistake, take it lightly; don't shame yourself. After all, even badass yoga teachers are human. Make any acknowledgment of a mistake with a swift lightheartedness that does not violate students' trust of you. I say *swift* because you should not dwell on the mishap—acknowledge it and move on. An apology is OK if you make it with confidence. If you are constantly apologizing with a nervous "Sorry, sorry, sorry," it is likely your students will lose their ability to have faith in your words and guidance. Again, the likelihood that they even notice the aspects of the class you would have liked to have done differently are slim.

Reflections:

Do you allow yourself to make mistakes as part of your growth process?

Do you take risks in your life choices? What happens when you do?

Before You Teach...

Kapalabhati is a vigorous breathing technique that can be used to stimulate manipura chakra. Often known as "skull-shining breath," *kapalabhati* comes from two Sanskrit words: *kapala*, which translates to "skull," and *bhati*, which means "light." It is a breathing technique that rejuvenates, purifies, and invigorates the mind and body. To perform kapalbhati, there is a focus on passive inhalation and active exhalation, where you inhale normally and exhale forcefully. With each exhalation, snap the belly in and up, breathing forcefully through the nose. The inhalations will happen naturally, so be sure to emphasize the forceful exhalation.

It is said that when this breath is practiced, your skull is filling with a bright light—hence the name. Kapalabhati breath helps gather the energy of the lower chakras upward into conscious awareness of the higher chakras. To deepen the connection to manipura chakra, bring the palms to rest on the solar plexus. Other benefits of kapalbhati breathing are:

- Improves digestion
- Reduces belly fat
- Strengthens and tones diaphragm and abdominal muscles
- Clears the mind and focuses attention
- Energizes the body by releasing toxins
- Cleanses lungs and respiratory system
- Increases oxygen to cells, purifying blood in the process
- Warms body

Poses for a Third-Chakra Sequence

1. Virabhadrasana 1 (warrior I)
2. Virabhadrasana 2 (warrior II)
3. Virabhadrasana 3 (warrior III)
4. Trikonasana (triangle pose)
5. Ardha Chandrasana (half-moon pose)
6. Utthita Parsvakonasana (extended side-angle pose)
7. Navasana (boat pose)
8. Purvottanasana (reverse plank pose)
9. Dhanurasana (bow-pulling pose)
10. Ardha Matsyendrasana (half lord of the fishes, seated twist pose)

Four

Have a Heart and Make Connections

*The way is not in the sky. The
way is in the heart.*

—*Buddha*

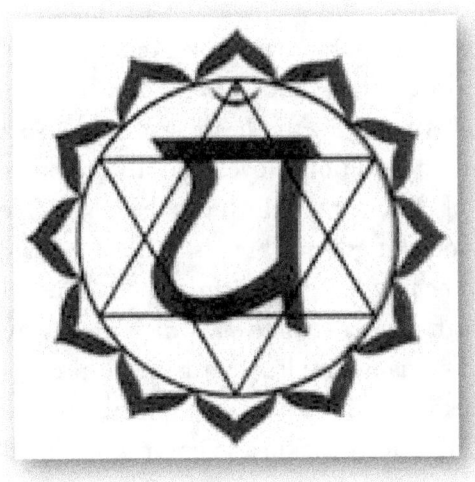

Chakra Four Overview

Name: Anahata (unstruck)
Element: Air
Color: Green
Purpose: Balance, love
Basic Rights: To love and be loved
Properties: Radiance, openness, expansion
Signs of Deficiency: Withdrawn, antisocial, prone to feelings of loneliness and depression, narcissism, general fear of relationships
Signs of Excess: Jealous, demanding of others, clingy, exhibits poor boundaries
Signs of Balance: Compassionate, loving, peaceful, balanced, empathetic to others
Demons: Grief, negativity

The fourth chakra is at the center of the seven chakras with three below and three above, but I like to think of Anahata as being in the heart center, the space of absolute joy and unconditional love. Since this chakra is located at the center of the chest and includes the heart, cardiac plexus, thymus gland, lungs, and breasts, it is often said to be the area where the physical and spiritual meet. The Sanskrit word for the fourth chakra is *anahata*, which means "unstruck" or "unhurt." The name implies that beneath the pain and grief of past experiences lies a pure and spiritual place where only bliss exists. The heart chakra also governs our interaction with the external world and regulates our feelings of compassion, love, and devotion. When the heart chakra is open, you are flowing with kindness, tolerance, and joy. You find it easy to forgive others who have caused you pain, and you are in a place of acceptance of yourself and others. A deficient heart chakra can cause strong emotions of anger, jealousy, grief, betrayal, and loathing toward yourself and others. A balanced heart chakra is exemplified in that you give in proportion to what we take, you can be vulnerable when in pain, and you are able to spread love when feeling joyful.

The heart chakra is a very popular focal point in many yoga classes. We all want to feel love, to share love with others, and to enjoy all the happiness, experiences, and magic moments that come with it. Yoga knows that we are beings of energy and that our body, heart, and mind are all aspects of the same vital life force. So when our heart and mind engage in asana practice, the heart and mind are also opened up and liberated accordingly. The sense associated with the heart chakra is touch. The organ is the skin, with emphasis on the hands, which communicate the loving healing power of anahata through hugs, massage, and touch. People who have awakened the heart chakra make great teachers and healers, due to the high level of loving energy and deep inner peace that emanates from them.

We can heal anahata by practicing forgiveness and understanding. Only when we forgive can we free our hearts to be open, so we can move forward. When we let go of our old hurts and pains, we can make room for more love to come into our lives. As you may recall from your own past experiences, forgiveness is not easy, and it often doesn't come naturally or willingly. When our suffering is strong, it is even harder to find the strength to forgive another. Remind yourself that forgiveness doesn't insinuate that the pain isn't or wasn't real or that what happened to you didn't matter. Rather, forgiveness opens you up to see the learning opportunity that difficult experiences can provide. When we can end the victim mentality, we can reclaim our lives, find acceptance, and move onward and upward.

Reflections:

What conditions do you put on yourself or others in order to be open to love?

Does forgiveness come easily for you?

How can your forgiveness benefit others?

Fourth Chakra Yoga-Teaching Tips

Create community. Even though yoga is a practice that suggests going within and finding the connection to ourselves, a little warmth and connection before class transforms the mood and begins the building of community. When teachers know students well and students know one another, the bonds begin to form for a strong community. To foster this sense of community and relationship building, be sure to introduce yourself at the beginning of class; when possible, make a special point to connect with those who are new to the practice or studio. Walking into an unfamiliar space can be a daunting experience, so you should do your best to always make students feel as welcomed and comfortable as possible. The intimate experience of feeling like you belong provides long-lasting benefits to anahata chakra. As I mentioned in chakra two, remember people's names, speak to them by name during class, and always thank people for the efforts they put into their practice.

Don't be cliquey. If you thought cliques were a thing of your past, something from your high school years, you thought wrong. Cliques are tightly knit groups of individuals who socialize and often exclude others, and this behavior occurs in yoga studios around the world. A close-knit group of students and teachers can appear exclusive and unwelcoming to outsiders, so always remember to reach out to new students and practitioners at the places you teach. Have you ever practiced at a studio that did not feel welcoming, or have you felt there were cliques that you were clearly not a part of? I have, and it is not a good feeling. Repeated feedback from customers at our studio locations involves the inclusive and familial feeling present from the moment they walk into the space. I attribute this vibe as a key factor in the success of the studio, and it is perpetuated by surrounding myself with teachers and staff who have the same core values as I do. Creating a sense of community touches the hearts of the students, and it is that heart-centered feeling that keeps people coming back to their mats. Play your part in cultivating that feeling.

Support other teachers in your community. Showing up on the mat is one of the easiest ways to show your appreciation for fellow teachers. Attending classes and supporting your community is a way of representing professionalism, collaboration, education, and appreciation of your local tribe. As badass yoga teachers, we should be all-inclusive, one tribe, regardless of style of yoga or studio affiliation. After all, yoga is inclusive.

There is always something to learn by practicing with different teachers, and when you practice at studios where you also teach, it does not go unnoticed. Most yoga studios' owners seem to feel that when teachers practice, it shows that they value the community and strive to be a part of it. Students will enjoy seeing you in the room with them, as it really validates the essence of the practice as an important part of a daily routine. Lead by example and embody the energy you want to receive. The more we see other teachers as resources, the more you can shift from the perspective of scarcity and into a perspective of being enough. The more interdependent you feel in your yoga community, the more badass you will become.

Seek a mentor. The role of a mentor is to encourage the personal and professional development of a mentee through the sharing of knowledge, expertise, and experience.

The mentoring relationship is built on mutual trust, respect, and communication and involves both parties meeting regularly to exchange ideas, discuss progress, and set goals for further growth. Develop a relationship with someone who inspires you on the yogic path, preferably someone who is also a teacher. Experienced teachers can deeply connect us to the lineage of the practice by transmitting the love and knowledge they have received from *their* mentors. Over time, a mentor will recognize your patterns (samskaras) and help to expose them. A mentor can notice little things about your practice and your teaching. This could be anything from bringing attention to your fidgeting in savasana, commenting on how you say "um" a lot in your teaching, or pointing out that you favor one shoulder in chaturanga. Regardless of your patterns, a teacher who sees you regularly will notice this and find a loving way to call it to your attention. This process helps to cultivate self-awareness and uncover the patterns that hold us back from our true selves and the potential we have on and off the mat. Find a mentor, make an effort to connect with that person often, and share both your victories and struggles. A mentor can also offer mutually beneficial support as you can learn from each other and hold each other accountable to perform at your highest potential.

Teach from love, even to the difficult students. If you want to be a strong influence for the students who show up in your classes, you need not only love to teach, though you should love each person you teach. Try to understand those you teach. I find that many teachers get overwhelmed by more difficult students or brand-new beginners who show up to their classes. No doubt beginners can be a challenge, as they come with a minimal frame of reference for the practice that can cause a new teacher to feel distracted or even annoyed. However, there are many lessons to be learned when teaching beginners. I like to remind myself that every time a newbie shows up, I have an opportunity to make them love yoga—or on the flip side, I can be responsible for them never stepping foot on their mat again. How is that for pressure? Therefore, you need to lead with love and compassion and be in a continual search for ways to help new students and those who have been less active feel welcome in your classes.

New teachers are often advised to teach beginner classes. There is a notion that these are the easiest classes to teach, but for me at least, they can be the hardest—albeit very rewarding. It is imperative that you let go of your perception of a "perfect class" when teaching any student, regardless of experience level. When you teach to beginners, it is likely that they have not been active in any fitness modality recently. You may encounter a significant percentage who have some kind of injury or sickness or who have a very superficial understanding of yoga, causing some to initially have a minimal receptivity to the practice. Always remember to be honest and straightforward, and make eye contact to show you care and want the best for them. After all, we were all beginners once.

Beginner or not, there will always be some students who just won't get what you are trying to explain, no matter how many times and in how many ways you explain and offer guidance. After a few tries without any notice of their receptivity, considering they are not about to hurt themselves, just let them be. You can't force or rush the process; this is their yoga practice more than it is your class. If you really follow the concept of fitting the yoga to the student and not the other way around, then every student should have a totally different-looking practice, according to his or her individual abilities, needs, and desires. In many yoga classes, especially in beginner classes, the pressure to "get it right" is sometimes way too big, and I feel that as a teacher, it is your responsibility to lessen the pressure and not to reinforce it. No matter how much alignment you study, in the end, there is no right and wrong in yoga. And that is a much more valuable lesson for students than perfecting all the details of every posture.

Practice unconditional compassion for all human beings, especially for the more difficult students. They are your greatest teachers, if you just change the way you think about them. We never know what someone else is bringing to their mat or why they need a yoga practice, so it is always best to handle all individuals with kindness, compassion, and care. When you offer guidance to a student, show compassion, even if he or she chooses to ignore your suggestions. If a student takes frequent breaks, struggles, grunts, or does other things that cause distractions in class, show them kindness and understanding, too. Your role as a teacher means you allow and foster individual expression and empowerment (think back to chakra three). How about the student who takes child's pose repeatedly? For many students, resting in class while others are pushing hard takes a lot of courage and letting go of ego. I sometimes explain that a pose like child's pose is very advanced, because it requires letting go of the competitive mind, or ego. So bravo to them! How about the student who gets up and leaves in the middle of class or, maybe even worse, before savasana? Students are coming to your class voluntarily, and as difficult as it may be at times, you also need to allow them to leave as they want. You give the challenges, but they're theirs to take or leave.

Now let's examine a slightly different take on teaching from love. You may have heard a quote similar to, "Do what you love, and the money will follow." There is no doubt that yoga has made it to the mainstream. Classes are held in health clubs and hospitals and during lunch hour in corporate buildings. Teaching yoga certainly seems safe and long-term as far as occupations go. Studies show there are full-time yoga teachers who are grossing more than $100,000 a year. A select few are making more than $200,000, although the majority gross $25,000 to $50,000.

Love what you do enough to do it well. Be committed. Be purposeful. Go into teaching for the love of the practice. If you become a yoga teacher with the desire for monetary wealth, you may become quickly discouraged and drained of your passion. I have seen it time and time again when a yoga teacher's salary becomes the main source of income; full-time yoga teachers become more stressed and attached to the fruits of their actions, and inevitably, they lose the love and passion that brought them into the role of the teacher. Yet I have met many yoga teachers who teach solely for the joy of teaching, who are not dependent on their getting paid as the main motivation for sharing the practice, and it is often those teachers who are more easily able to sustain the passion that drove them into the field of teaching.

To be a yoga teacher, you must be in a position where self-employment can be an option. If you have dependents or a lot of debt, self-employment can seem very scary and perhaps too risky. Do not lose heart, but you will have to proceed more cautiously. I always tell new teachers during teacher training, "Don't quit your day jobs yet!" Start slowly, with one or two classes per week. Teaching with love is not easy, but we all know nothing of importance is. Like any other profession, teaching yoga calls for a particular set of skills, talent, and drive. If you are in it for the long haul, with true passion for the practice and the desire to share the wonderful benefits to others, it will be the toughest job you will ever love.

Offer Adjustments. There are always opportunities, even with intermediate and advanced students, to help them have a deeper experience. Assisting students is a great way to inspire them to open, expand, and release tension. The quickest way to get students to *not* come back to your class is to ignore them. Students choose a class setting versus watching an online video because they want a connection. Sometimes even the smallest adjustment to a student's position in a posture will make a huge difference in his or her overall experience. Just because a student is doing well in a posture does not mean he or she won't benefit from your help. There are many reasons teachers offer assists and adjustments and many things that over time your teacher eye will recognize. Here are a few guidelines on what or why assists can help:

- To remove student from an unsafe position that could potentially lead to injury
- To give energetic information about a pose
- To increase a student's awareness of his or her body or breath
- To provide alternative ways of experiencing and/or deepening the pose
- To offer encouragement
- To respond to a student who is asking for guidance or clarification
- To give a student a "feel good adjustment" that helps to deepen, stretch, or massage

There are a few specific danger zones that a badass teacher should be aware of. Use extreme care with the cervical spine, the lower back and the S.I. (sacroiliac) joint. Never put pressure directly on the spine in any assist. Notice the foundation of the pose, which is always what is on the ground. Usually the foundation is one's feet, but the foundation of a pose can involve hands, forearms, or even the head, depending on the pose. Notice common danger signs, like knees going over toes in warrior I or warrior II or shoulders cranked up by the ears in standing postures. These are positions that should catch your eye for some needed attention.

If a student is very flexible, especially if their joints hyperextend, then focus your adjustments on reiterating their foundation and connecting them to their core strength. To avoid taking the student out of balance, you must first feel stable in your own posture. I recommend being in a lunge, horse stance, or squat as a conducive stance for physical adjusting. Your own stability can be the key to making the adjustment feel safe, efficient, and effective for the student. If you feel any resistance from the student, stop and observe. Err on the side of caution, always.

Often in teacher training, I suggest that physical assists should be done primarily on students you know, whose practice you are familiar with. Then there is a better understanding of how that particular body can be approached most safely and effectively. When you wish to practice a cool new assist you just learned at a workshop, or perhaps a juicy assist you were lucky enough to experience in your own body, I would suggest practicing with a peer (a fellow yoga teacher) first, before using students and paying customers as your guinea pigs. By practicing with a fellow teacher, you can receive valuable and informed feedback that can allow you the opportunity to refine your touch for your students.

I also acknowledge that not all teacher trainings place a strong emphasis on physical assists; some focus attention more on verbal cues. If you are not trained or confident in physical assists in the role of teacher, then find a continuing-education workshop or a teacher who can oversee you. It is the only way to ensure we are being guided with the least amount of potential harm to our students. Start small; work on mastering one particular assist at a time, building your repertoire slowly and effectively. Remember that yoga is a practice of process, not attainment. The same goes for teaching! Enjoy the unique-ness, beauty, and oneness of all who step foot in your class. Strive to have the students feel freer in their bodies and their breath, as that is the highest form of yoga we can offer.

In order to safely adjust students, it is important to know if any of the students have pertinent past or present injuries that may present themselves in the postures or if the students are pregnant or have other relevant conditions. In addition, in order for students to feel comfortable opting out of adjust-ments for any reason at all, giving them the confidential option before class is a good strategy. I suggest having the students in a child's pose or position that is inward to allow for some privacy. Some teachers have students place stones, sticky notes, or other indicators on their mats to indicate their choice to have or not have adjustments.

Be aware of the energy. Much of the benefit of Hatha yoga is the effect the practice has on the "energy body." Improvements in alignment, stability, and flexibility remove obstacles to free physical energy flow. So from this perspec-tive, we might consider any assists we provide as "energetic," in the sense that there is no real separation between physical and energetic bodies. We experience them as directly related. Through their exploration of the body and breath, the ancient yogis discovered that prana (life force energy) could be further subdivided into energetic components, called vayus (winds). The five vayus of prana all have very subtle yet distinct ener-getic qualities, including specific functions and directions of flow, and this energetic flow is represented in yoga asana. As teachers, as did the ancient yogis, we can help students cultivate these vayus by simply bringing focus and awareness to them within the practice. Giving students even a basic awareness of one or more of the vayus will help them deepen their body and breath awareness, which will enrich their entire yoga practice.

Prana-Vayu is situated in the head, centered in the third-eye, and its energy pervades the chest region. The flow of Prana-Vayu is upward. It nourishes the brain and eyes and governs reception of all things: food, air, senses, and thoughts. In the yoga postures, the flow of prana-vayu exists in which body parts present the highest point. For example, in Tadasana (mountain pose), prana-vayu would be rising out of the head.

Apana-vayu interplays with prana-vayu as it is generally in the opposite position; in Tadasana, for example, apana would be in the feet, as a grounding or rooting-down energy. Apana-vayu is situated in the pelvic floor, and its energy pervades the lower abdomen. As this energy is downward and out, apana-vayu nourishes the organs of digestion, reproduction, and elimination. Apana-vayu governs the elimination of all substances from the body: carbon monoxide, urine, stool, menstrual blood, and so on.

Vyana-vayu is situated in the heart and lungs and flows throughout the entire body. The flow of vyana-vayu moves from the center of the body to the periphery, so in the yoga postures, this presents itself through the limbs. In Tadasana, vyana-vayu is seen through the arms being active and the fingers ignited. It governs circulation of all substances throughout the body and assists the other vayus with their functions.

Udana-vayu is situated in the throat and has a circular flow around the neck and head. It functions to "hold us up" and governs speech, self-expression, and growth. This vayu is less present in yoga postures but can represent itself in breath and sweat. The postures that exude udana-vayu most clearly are poses that allow the throat to be open, such as Ustrasana (camel pose) or Urdhva Dhanurasana (upward-facing bow).

Samana-vayu is situated in the abdomen with its energy centered in the navel. The flow of samana-vayu moves from the periphery of the body to the center. In Tadasana, samana can be evident through the squeezing in of the navel and inner thighs. Samana-vayu governs the digestion of all substances: food, air, experiences, emotions, and thoughts.

I find the awareness of where the energy flows (vayus) in postures to be very helpful to increase the eye of the teacher, particularly when deciding on physical assists that could be beneficial for the student. When observing a student, ask yourself: Does he or she need more grounding in the pose (apana)? What can use more lift (prana)? What can be more centered and squeezed in (samana)? Are all body parts reaching and expressed in the posture (vyana)? Is he or she breathing (udana)?

Instruct Pranayama. Breathing is a vital function of life. In yoga, we refer to conscious breathing as pranayama. *Prana* is a Sanskrit word that means life force, and *ayama* means extending or stretching. Thus, the word *pranayama* translates to the control of life force. It is also known as the extension of breath. Every cell in the body needs oxygen to function properly, so it's no surprise that research shows that a regular practice of controlled breathing can decrease the effects of stress on the body and increase overall physical and mental health.

As the element of chakra four is air, we can relate anahata chakra to breath, a giving and receiving of air, or even a giving and receiving of love. Breath is essential to life, as it is the first thing we do when we are born and the last thing we do when we die. In between that time, we take about half a billion breaths. However, without a mindful yoga practice, you may not pay attention to many breaths; the air may just go in and out without any consciousness of it. Yet yoga helps us to realize that the mind, body, and breath are intimately connected and have strong influences on one another. Learning to breathe consciously and with awareness can be a valuable tool in helping to restore balance in the mind and body, and as yoga teachers, it is our job to incorporate breath work, or pranayama, as part of the practice. It is an essential limb of the eightfold path and should not be ignored. Researchers have documented the benefits of a pranayama practice. Some of the benefits are:

- Decreased feelings of stress and being overwhelmed
- Reduced feelings of anxiety and depression
- Lowered and more stabilized blood pressure
- Boosts in energy levels
- Increased muscle relaxation

Conscious breathing also connects us to the third sheath, mano-maya kosha, or mind sheath. This kosha involves the functions of the mind that relate to everyday living and our individual interpretation and experience of life. The manomaya kosha can be either useful or detrimental, depending on how we train the mind. Fortunately, the practice of yoga is designed to bring out the higher functions of manomaya kosha, and pranayama is a useful tool in calming the mind. Yoga teaches us that when the breath is erratic, the mind is erratic. Control of the breath is instrumental in balancing annamaya kosha, pranamaya kosha, and manomaya kosha combined.

Teach with vulnerability. The process of being vulnerable is an expression of your humanity and gives others permission to feel whatever they need to feel on the mat. Have you ever heard the term *the issues are in the tissues*? Have you ever experienced or witnessed an emotional breakthrough during a yoga practice or a cry of release or even joy in savasana? If so, then you know what I am talking about! Being vulnerable does not imply that you use your role as a teacher to over-share about your personal life or that you have no boundaries with students. To the contrary, it invites you to express your authentic journey through yoga and yoga teaching as a muse to illuminate the path for others. If you teach with a huge wall up around you, your students will be able to feel it. You've got to be open in order to create a space for true transformation to occur. Vulnerability fosters trust and honest communication, so when you are vulnerable as a teacher, students will be more likely to be open and vulnerable with you.

Being vulnerable means having the ability to connect and listen fully, without being caught up in your own mental chatter and without making what they say be about *you*. This act of being vulnerable requires you to admit that you don't know everything, so you can be open and present in the moment. Your vulnerability won't just be of benefit to the students you teach but will also teach you a great deal about yourself as well. It means fully showing up for the students and accepting that you will not have all the answers. It is the ability to say what needs to be said, even if the student might have a hard time hearing it. Vulnerability is allowing yourself to be seen, as sometimes the gift of your open presence is the most powerful gift you can give students.

Learn to Share. The greatest gift of having knowledge is the ability to share this knowledge with others. In yoga, there is no "yours" or "mine." Let go of the thoughts that other teachers are stealing your sequences or ideas, and make peace with a sharing of inspiration instead. Create a mentality built on abundance and practice nonattachment. It is a beautiful thing to take a class and be inspired to later share a flow, sequence, or quote that you experienced with another teacher. And imitation is a great expression of admiration, so even if a teacher "steals" your sequence, the exciting thing about being a yoga teacher is that no one can be you. Even if someone were to use your exact words, the experience would still never be the same as when you taught it. Honor the uniqueness of who you are as a teacher. Consider giving kudos to those who inspire you. Express your yoga teachings freely, without agenda or need for accolades for your offerings. Remember, the opposite of sharing is stealing.

The Demon of Negativity

As the center of our emotional intelligence, any imbalance occurring in anahata may give way to negative thoughts and feelings. Yoga is a practice that meets you where you are and allows you the freedom to choose your response. Patanjali teaches us that "When disturbed by negative thoughts, opposite (positive) ones should be thought of instead" (*Vitarka badhane pratipaksha bhavana,* Sutra 2.33). Basically, this suggests that when we control the mind and obstruct the thoughts we do not want, we invite in the opposite thoughts. If you can remind yourself of this sutra, you will see your whole reality change rather quickly.

Reflections:

Identify three ways you can shift negative thinking.

Are there times you feel like not being happy? What do you think causes this?

Before You Teach...

As the color associated with the heart chakra is green, be green. Go outside in nature as much as you can; even wearing more green clothing can instill more love and compassion into your teaching and your way of being. The heart chakra is associated with the vibrational sound of YAM. Chant this before you teach or whenever you feel yourself closing your heart to the world or having difficulty leading with love.

Poses for a Fourth-Chakra Sequence

1. Gomukhasana (cow face pose)
2. Marjaryasana and Bitilasana (cat and cow poses)
3. Anahatasana (puppy dog pose)
4. Matsyasana (fish pose)
5. Ustrasana (camel pose)
6. Urdhva Dhanurasana (upward-facing bow pose)
7. Adho Mukha Vrksasana (handstand)
8. Camatkarasana (wild thing pose)
9. Natarajasana (lord of the dancer's pose)

Five

USE YOUR VOICE AND BE CREATIVE

*We have two ears and one mouth so that
we can listen twice as much as we speak.*

—*EPICTETUS*

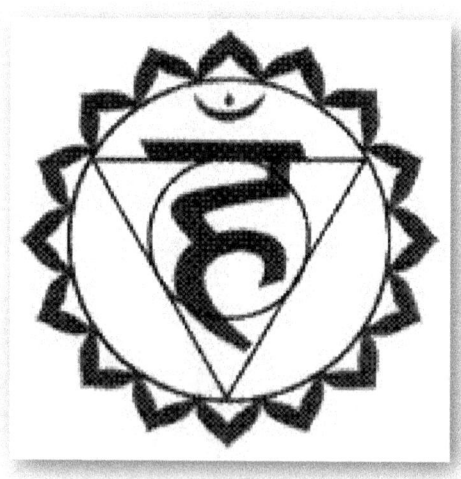

Chakra Five Overview

Name: Vishuddha (purification)
Element: Ether
Color: Bright blue
Purpose: Communication, creativity
Basic Right: To be heard
Properties: Creativity, harmony, coherence, truth
Signs of Deficiency: Difficulty putting thoughts into words, fear of speaking, excessive shyness
Signs of Excess: Talking too much or inappropriately, gossiping, inability to keep secrets
Signs of Balance: Full and resonant voice, good communication skills with others, good listener, sense of timing and rhythm
Demon: Gossip

The fifth chakra, Vishuddha, is the first of the three spiritual chakras and is located in the throat region. It governs the anatomical regions of the thyroid, parathyroid, jaw, neck, mouth, tongue, and larynx. With its placement between the fourth and sixth chakras, a balanced throat center facilitates harmony between the heart and the head. When vishuddha is excessive, a person often interrupts and talks over others and is generally not a good listener. When the fifth chakra is deficient, the voice is soft and/or unsteady, and the person may be shy and introverted. Another indication of throat-chakra imbalance is tone deafness and an inability to distinguish the pitch and tonal quality of one's own voice. To be open and balanced in the fifth chakra, one has the ability to speak, listen, and express oneself freely and doesn't doubt or question one's own words or voice. For badass yoga teachers, having a clear voice plays a vital role in our ability to communicate with students.

The fifth chakra represents your creative identity, based on the ways you express yourself. It is the realm of consciousness that creates, controls, transmits, and receives communication with ourselves and others, as it moves our inner thoughts outward into the world. Chakra five is at the forefront of creating something new and includes listening, speaking, chanting, writing, and the arts. Yoga asana, pranayama, and mantra practice can open, stimulate, and purify vishuddha chakra and penetrate and release the emotional blocks or struggles we feel. The practice has the potential to release this energy, and then quite spontaneously, we begin to understand ourselves at a deeper level; we can understand and express the inner truth of a situation, being clearer about what we feel and what we really need. After this higher level of self-realization in awakening vishuddha, the Spirit is able to interact with our consciousness much more clearly and directly. When the fifth chakra awakens, we become blessed with a greater power to communicate and influence others. Because of the chakra's ability to transform events and experiences into joy, a person with balance in vishuddha can lead by example in order to teach and inspire others to greater change.

Metaphysics of the Hindu culture believe everything in the universe is made of sound. Within everything is a symbolic representation of its particular energy pattern, often called a seed sound or *bija* mantra. Chanting the sounds or bijas is said to create resonance with the object of the sound. Within each human being lies the power to affect change through the power of a chant, the spoken words, or even a gentle whisper. The body's chakras or energy centers, so closely intertwined with their corresponding regions of the body, can be represented in sound, which parallels the energy pattern of the chakras and is symbolic of their essences. These unique sounds are the bija, or seed, mantras. The mantras are the one-syllable seed sounds that, when said aloud, activate the energy of the chakras in order to purify and balance the mind and body. When you speak the bija mantras, you resonate with the energy of the associated chakra, helping you focus upon your own instinctive awareness of your body and its needs. OM is the most renowned and expensive of the bija mantras. It is the mantra of creation, and its chant causes energy to surge upward and outward. In traditional Hatha Yoga, there are seven bija mantras associated with the chakras:

1. LAM for the earth chakra
2. VAM for the water chakra
3. RAM for the fire chakra
4. YAM for the heart chakra
5. HAM for the throat chakra
6. AUM or OM for the third eye
7. No mantra for the crown chakra, so the bija is silence

The following is a list of commonly used mantras and their meanings. This list is small in comparison to the number of mantras that exist, but you may find these effective.

Lokah samastha sukhino bhavanthu

May all beings be happy and free from suffering.

Gayatri Mantra

(Perhaps the most revered of all Hindu mantras, this is found in the *Rig-Veda* (62.62).

Om bhur bhuvah svaha
Thath savitur varenyam
Bhargo dheyvasya dhimahih
Dhyoyonah pratchodhay-yath

We worship the word that is present in the earth, the heavens, and that which is beyond. By meditating on this glorious power that gives us life, we ask that our minds and hearts be illuminated.

Om Namah Shivaaya

Om Namah Shivaaya, Namah Shivaaya, Namah Shiva
I bow to Lord Shiva, the peaceful one who is the embodiment of all that is caused by the universe.

So Hum

(Designed to unite the individual with the universe)
I am that; that I am.

Reflections:

Are there instances where you feel you do not have the right to speak or be heard?

Are there circumstances where you feel you speak but are not heard?

Fifth Chakra Yoga-Teaching Tips

Use Your Voice. The pace of your voice defines the rhythm of the class and can influence how your students breathe. Pay special attention to the way the class is moving. For example, do you notice a majority of the class is moving behind your cues? This may be an indication that their breath integration with movement is a bit slower than your words. Slow it down! If you are cueing too fast, it may be harder for your students to go inward. Enjoy this opportunity to be connected with your students and adjust your pace accordingly. A general rule is that 80 percent of the class should be moving with your cues. There will always be those few who are moving beyond your words and a few lagging behind, but if you can gauge about 80 percent of the class following along, your pacing is on the right track.

The tone, pitch, volume, and inflection of your voice really do matter. When you speak in a monotone or as quietly as a mouse, how do you expect anyone to be motivated to follow along? It also becomes increasingly difficult to keep the mind focused when the engagement and passion of the teacher, as presented through his or her voice, is lacking. On the same note, students may want to relax. After a hard day of work, the last thing they want to hear is a drill sergeant's voice barking commands at them. Like all things in yoga, there should be a balance in your voice: a firmness that suggests you are confident and students can trust your guidance but also a gentleness and awareness that allow students to be comfortable and calm. The inflection in your cueing can create a different emphasis and touch a different emotion and energetic quality. A skilled teacher can use his or her voice to regain a student's attention and can use vocal rhythm to dictate when a pose should be energetic or restful.

Practice saying less. Perhaps Einstein said it best: "make things as simple as possible, but not simpler." I am not suggesting you leave out pertinent information that could help students get deeper; rather, consider eliminating words that do not add value to your teaching. Let your instructions be fluid and informed but not overly complex. Every asana has at least a few dozen points about position, alignment, energy, and effort. Common weaknesses with newer teachers are that they say too many of these points, say not enough of them, or choose the ones that aren't necessary. One way to give the perfect amount of instruction is to observe the students and use them as a guide to what needs to be said. See what they need to hear, and cue from that. When we teach only the poses, but don't teach them to the people who are actually in the room, we are wasting time and energy. Speaking to what you see makes each instruction more potent. It is also a reiteration of being present, a manifestation of the first of Patanjali's yoga sutras, which states, "Yoga is now."

Notice if you add unnecessary words into your cues, and if you do, try to eliminate those extra words from your instruction. Words and phrases such as "um," "now go ahead…" and "now we are gonna…" are fillers that offer no help to your students and take up precious time. When you offer cues to the class, think "verb, body part, direction." For example, you might say, "Reach your arms overhead," or "Step your feet to the front of your mat." Being as concise as possible with your words is a sure way to have the class moving more effortlessly inward.

Be on the lookout for signs of confusion or students who need frequent visual direction. Change your language as needed, but know that at times you may need to provide a visual to demonstrate a position that is not being understood via your words. Use those opportunities to reflect on what you can do differently next time you cue that sequence or pose. Take every opportunity to grow into a more badass yoga teacher.

Embrace the power of OM. I encourage you to celebrate the spiritual aspects of this practice with your students, and in doing so, find the words that help tap into their innate understanding of oneness and the presence of divinity. You may begin to see that this magic will make students keep coming to your classes. If all you offer in your teaching is the mindset of getting a thin yoga body and a handstand, then you will only be offering a surface level of yoga to your students. Yes, it is true that offering a yoga practice for merely the health benefits will result in practitioners feeling better, having more energy, and enjoying improved overall health. But this is not the depth the practice can allow. In order to really get the deepest benefit from the practice, you have to offer an intention on the spiritual journey of yoga. If you know your reason for doing the practice is to be a more peaceful, patient, and happy person, then all the necessary lessons that lead to that result will become evident within the practice.

We are conditioned to avoid pain and attach to pleasure. There will be constant obstacles thrown in your way to disturb your peace; such as traffic, bills, or a broken appliance. Yoga is not about getting rid of all these experiences with a desire to take control of our external environments; in fact, it is quite the opposite. Yoga is about keeping your peace of mind regardless of whether you experience ease and joy or stress and pain. Attempting to change your external situations is a battle sure to be lost. Instead, teach your students that learning to gain control of their thoughts and reactions is something way more worth mastering than a handstand. Strive to take your students to this deeper level in your teaching. You will be playing an integral role in making the world a more peaceful place.

There are many ways you can invite and engage the spiritual aspects of yoga into a class, and the term "God" doesn't have to be mentioned at all. In fact, a simple chant of OM is enough to embrace the divine. In fact, the word *OM* represents everything. It is said to be the seed of all creation.

This seemingly small word contains all the power of the universe—it is the beginning, middle, and end or the past, present, and future. OM has vast popularity simply because of its vibration, which is felt not only within the room when it's chanted, but which is created in the body. The sound is known to soothe the nervous system almost immediately. It has the ability to remove mind chatter and prepares us to be more receptive and contemplative. In a class setting, it really does unite the group and creates a sense of togetherness and community. Chanting a unified OM aligns the bodies, minds, and spirits of the practitioners to become more as one. It is a grounding and peaceful sound that may be enough to set a spiritual tone to your classes.

Speak from what you know. When you teach, remind yourself that you are talking to people. While it's true that we do teach poses, and some days our teaching is more on point than others, we are always teaching those things to human beings. Consider something that you know very well, like how to wash your hair. It would probably be very easy for you to teach that to somebody, and your words would be clear, sequential, and specific. There is no reason to speak any differently or put on a *teacher voice*, because you are speaking from what you know. Assuming you know what you are teaching, this strategy opens up communication in familiar territory, which helps you teach effectively in and with your own voice.

In teacher training, I am often asked whether it's OK to teach things you can't necessarily do yourself. The answer is yes and no. Some schools of thoughts on this topic suggest that if it's something you can't do because you have a broken arm, then yes, it's fine to teach this, assuming you were able to do it before breaking your arm. Otherwise, no—why would you want to teach something you don't know? I speak to many teachers, and often there is a feeling of pressure—an idea that, as yoga teachers, we must get to the next advanced pose. In yoga practice, the work is meant to point our minds to the perfect present, not to the future that hasn't already occurred. Instead, try to use your practice and teaching as time to let go of the pressure to move on.

I do have some exceptions to this rule. Say a student would like to learn a forearm stand (pincha mayurasana) and asks you to teach him or her. You have not mastered that pose in your own practice—for the purpose of this discussion, mastering would mean you can hold a forearm stand unassisted for fifteen calm breaths. Even though you haven't mastered it, forearm stand is a pose that you do incorporate into your asana repertoire. Although you can't nail the pose every time or hold it for fifteen breaths, you know the foundation of the posture. You are clear on the alignment of the forearms, elbows, and wrists. You know that placing a block in the L shape of your fingers is a great use of the prop, as is using a strap for your upper arms. You know where the gaze should be and where the energy should flow. You are aware that kicking up with a strong, straight leg and squared hips will get you into the pose sooner. Then yes, you can guide a student into that pose, as you have explored it fully and repeatedly and have experienced the energy of the pose in your own body. If you teach a pose that you only aspire to acquire one day or a posture you've done only a few times, it will likely be ineffective teaching. Don't be discouraged; while there may be many things you aren't ready to teach, the flip side is that there are many things you do know very well and that your students would love to learn from you. Teach them those things.

Be authentic. No matter what we are doing, we do it better when we operate from an authentic space, and being a yoga teacher is no exception. Living from a place of authenticity means being rooted in your deepest beliefs, values, and truth and living a life that is a true reflection of them. It is about being true to yourself through your thoughts, words, and actions. It means being willing to sacrifice relationships, situations, or circumstances that violate your truth. For example, if you are in a relationship or profession that requires you to function in a way that is not in accord with your truth, you should leave it. Is this any easy task? No. However, you will have the wisdom of knowing who you are to guide you. The more you practice listening to your inner wisdom, the less friction and discontent you will find yourself creating in your life.

How can you be your most authentic self? It relies largely on where you place your focus. By holding the intention of being true to yourself, you focus your attention on whatever resonates with your truth. Through clear intentions and inner awareness, you begin to hold yourself accountable. Through discipline and commitment, you learn to do your best to live according to who you know yourself to be. That's profound authenticity.

You will inevitably embody the qualities of the teachers who have trained and influenced you, as you will teach the way the practice has been transmitted. However, teachers often feel pressured to eat perfectly or to embody the stereotype of a yoga teacher (whatever that means). But yoga teachers are people, too. Sometimes we drink too much, eat processed foods, have dysfunctional relationships, and act like fools. Dare I say *so what*? Students don't want or expect you to be perfect, but they do expect you to practice what you preach. If you teach an intense, sweaty ninety-minute hot yoga class but never practice hot, sweaty yoga, you're not teaching from an authentic place. If you teach a mindful-meditation class but don't have a meditation practice aside from when you're teaching, your students will see right through you. If you preach veganism but are seen out eating a hamburger, then people will notice and question your words thereafter. If what you are teaching doesn't feel authentic coming out of your mouth, then it probably shouldn't.

You don't need to have an advanced asana practice or ten million Instagram followers to be powerful, but you need to be dedicated to the practice and teach with authenticity. Anything less than 100 percent commitment will be seen as fake from a mile away, and you'll find yourself feeling drained and disingenuous as a teacher. Badass teaching is not stardom, and it's not easy or glamorous, but for teachers sharing from an authentic place, it can be the most rewarding path of doing what you love.

Encourage self-reflection. Elevate Vishuddha energy by giving students the opportunity to contemplate and connect to their truest and deepest understanding of self. If you're like most people, chances are you have questioned yourself: *Why do I always do that? Say that? Act like that? Think like that?* Whether they be losing your temper, taking on too much, or having negative self-talk, we all have some tendencies that are not serving us in a positive way. At times it can feel like these tendencies are just a part of who we are, but they aren't; they are habits and conditions that can be changed—albeit not always easily.

> *Samskara saksat karanat purvajati jnanam*
> *Through sustained focus and meditation on*
> *our patterns, habits, and conditioning, we*
> *gain knowledge and understanding of our past*
> *and of how we can change the patterns that*
> *aren't serving us to live more freely and fully.*

—*YOGA SUTRA 3.18*

In the above Sutra, Patanjali explains that samskaras, which are patterns or habits, can be a tool to refine the mind and come to a place of clearer perception. Samskaras are the subtle impressions of our past actions. The prefix *sam* means well planned and well thought out, and *kara* means "the action undertaken." Thus, *samskara* means "the impression of, the impact of, the action we perform with full awareness of its goals." When we perform such an action, a subtle impression is deposited into our minds. Each time the action is repeated, the impression becomes stronger. This is how a habit is formed. The stronger the habit, the less mastery we have over our mind when we try to execute an action that is not in accordance with our habitual patterns. Although Samskaras can be positive, negative, or neutral, the Samskaras that Patanjali is concerned with are the ones that affect our behavior negatively. As yoga teachers, it is our responsibility to bring to light some of these patterns that students may not even have awareness of. It is only through reflection that one can see the habits that hold us back and give the feeling of being stuck. It is as if you are presenting a mirror to your students, so they can see more clearly, get unstuck, and find the strength to move forward. It can seem like a daunting task, but as teachers of yoga, we are often very instrumental in guiding students through learning and reflection that create massive transformations in their lives.

Please use your words wisely. People are practicing yoga to get to a better place and be their best selves. They've chosen to take your class because they think you might help them do that. Remind yourself that you made the choice to teach so they could practice. Speak words that allow the practice to unfold without instilling criticism or judgment. As yoga teachers, we need to be mindful of not only our physical assists that may cause harm if not done properly but also of our language. We must refrain from using words toward our students that are condescending or that may create a sense of negative self-worth. For example, instead of saying, "If you're not flexible, bend your knees," we can simply say, "Bend your knees if it feels right," or, "if it's available, straighten the legs." Our goal on the path of teaching yoga is one of empowerment and strength. We want our students to realize their potential, not be told they are inflexible or not strong enough, or too big or too small, to achieve benefit from a posture. I encourage you all to be conscious at all times of your words when in the role of the teacher…and really, as an individual in this world, through all your interactions.

The Demon of Gossip

The demon of vishuddha chakra is any speech that carries a negative vibration out into the world, and there are few vibrations worse than gossip. In fact, even the yogic text Hatha Yoga Pradipika (1:15) states that "talkativeness" and "gossip" are destroyers of yoga and should be avoided. As a yoga teacher, you may bear witness to gossip or may be knee-deep in the trenches of it. Get out of the conversation! Or better yet, elevate the vibration by being an active optimist, conversation changer, or even giver of a reality check to those around you. Take the high road and offer a new perspective when negative talk is happening in your presence.

Reflection:

As a child, were there lies told in your family that you had to uphold? If so, how did that make you feel?

Before You Teach...

Sing a song! On your way to teach, sing a song in the car, hum down the street, or recite an OM Japa (repetition of OM)—anything to get your voice vibrations out into the universe. This will more easily connect you to the energy circulating in and around you and will help to clear any congestion in your voice before you teach.

Poses for a Fifth-Chakra Sequence

1. Parivrtta Parsvakonasana (revolved side-angle pose)
2. Bakasana (crane pose)
3. Sasangasana (rabbit pose)
4. Salamba Sarvangasana (shoulder-stand pose)
5. Halasana (plow pose)
6. Karnapidasana (ear pressure pose)

Six

BE INTUITIVE

In the depth of winter, I finally learned that within me there lay an invincible summer.

—*ALBERT CAMUS*

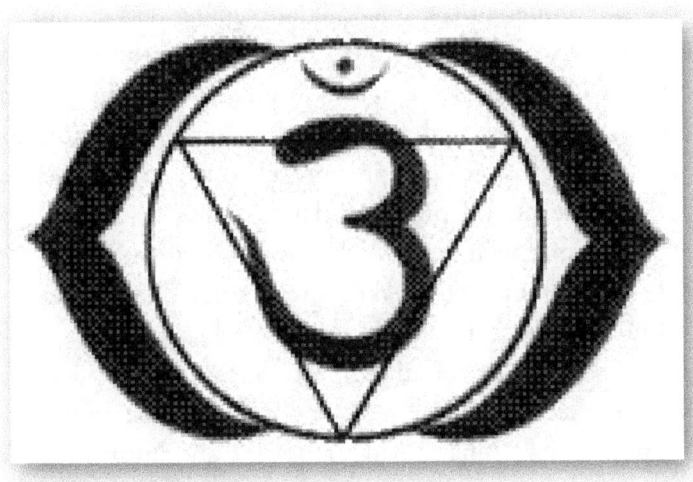

Chakra Six Overview

Name: Ajna (to perceive)
Element: Light
Color: Indigo
Purpose: Pattern recognition
Basic Rights: To see, to command
Properties: Radiance, single-pointed focus, steadiness
Signs of Deficiency: Difficulty visualizing, denial of circumstances, lack of imagination
Signs of Excess: Prone to delusions and/or hallucinations, frequent nightmares, difficulty with concentration
Signs of Balance: Creative imagination, ability to visualize, strong intuitive sense
Demon: Doubt

The journey of the chakra is now going deeper into the inner world. The sixth chakra, ajna, is in the area of the third eye or center of the brow. Although ajna is an invisible third eye, it is the highly powerful center of intuition and home to our visions and dreams. This chakra is associated with the pineal and pituitary glands and is responsible for hormonal management, which has a strong influence over body functioning. This chakra is responsible for imagination and higher levels of consciousness, so when in excess, difficulty concentrating and disconnection from reality can occur. When deficient, ajna can cause a faulty memory, headaches, and poor vision. Ajna provides a psychic and intuitive ability that allows for a "knowing of something" without being able to prove it, though it can felt with a gut instinct. People with a highly developed ajna chakra can have psychic gifts, such as having the ability to be highly sensitive to another person's thoughts and feelings.

By going into a state of meditation, turning consciousness away from the external world and inward, the mind is made quiet and open to receive the truth and insights available through the medium of ajna chakra. Ida and Pingala (female and male) channels arise from the root chakra and wrap around the central channel, Sushumna, to help form the main chakras at various points along the spine. They finally come together and finish their ascent in ajna chakra situated at the third eye. The main aim of yoga is to eventually unite these two forces at ajna chakra and achieve liberation from the suffering of duality and our mental habits of attachment to the world of the outward senses.

The outcome of the sixth chakra is to essentially work through your dreams and fantasies to create your own personal vision. It is through seeking ways of transcending our difficulties and challenges that we can become of service of others and be in the act of yoga. Your visions need to be on a macro scale, as well as a micro scale. It is through your intuition that you can expand your possibilities in your relationships, community, and work environment. It reminds us that, even through the difficult times, we should seek positive visions and aspirations for the goals we hope to achieve in creating the life we want.

Entering into the upper chakras moves us toward stillness. There is less emphasis on vigorous, athletic yoga asanas in the upper chakras but more emphasis on slowing your mind and body in preparation for meditation. It is in the third eye that you start to experience the union of mind and body and of the individual with the universe. We need to be still in order to see clearly. Let's take a look at the yoga sutras for some insight:

Now begins the instruction of yoga.

—SUTRA 1:1

*The restraint of the modification
of the mind-stuff is Yoga.*

—SUTRA 1:2

These first two verses of the yoga sutras imply several important ideas. First, we see an emphasis on *Now*. Yoga occurs in the present moment, not as much as a concept, but rather as a profound experience. Secondly, the reference to "instruction" calls upon the instruction being passed from teacher to student. It is so important to find a teacher with whom one can have a comfortable, trusting relationship and whose knowledge one respects. It is likely that students will need to go to a few teachers and experience a few different styles of yoga before it becomes clear which teacher speaks to them most. Lastly, and perhaps most useful, as this one concept describes all other sutras, is that the goal of yoga is to calm the mind chatter, the fluctuations of the mind-stuff. Essentially, we should be less distracted, more present, and still. When this is achieved, our true selves can be revealed.

Reflections:

What are you working on for the greater good of the world?

Where do you see possibilities that do not yet exist?

Sixth Chakra Yoga-Teaching Tips

Remain a student. I have mentioned this before, but I feel so strongly about the correlation to continuing your education and being a badass yoga teacher that I will discuss it again. A two hundred-hour program is only the icing on the cake, the tip of the iceberg of all yoga has to teach. This is a lifetime's practice, as both a teacher and a student. The sixth chakra is responsible for intellectual thinking and higher learning, so I recommend teachers practice different styles of yoga as part of their regimen, particularly those practices that challenge them to think in different ways. This can mean practicing yin, even though you teach vinyasa, or it can mean some days your practice is strictly pranayama instead of asana. There are many paths, as well as styles of yoga, that are all seeking to get you closer to bliss. Be sure to attend workshops and teacher trainings as often as possible to expand your wealth of knowledge and explore different components of teaching a yoga class. There is always something to take with you from maintaining a practice, whether it's a cue that resonated with you or a sequence that felt amazing. Or it can be the opposite: noticing what you didn't like and being sure to learn from that as well. Keep a connection to the work of the spiritual texts and the yoga masters before us; they are as accessible as we think they are. Remaining a student is an important part of being a clear and inspiring yoga teacher; it's so important that it's part of Yoga Alliance's requirements for registered yoga teachers.

Without the consideration of yourself as a student, the ego can easily take over and cause you to think you have all the answers. Continuing to learn from other teachers is a sure way to learn that you're not a perfect yogi, and other styles and interpretations can be just as wonderful as what you teach. It is also valuable to experience other teachers and teachings to learn what you don't like and how you don't want to be as a teacher. It's important to remain a student, because it gives you a greater perspective on the overall practice of yoga. It gives you a chance to learn new things and be in a state of awareness, reflection, and deeper understanding.

The struggle to maintain your own practice as a yoga teacher is very real. You may have to get really creative with ways you can fit the practice in. That is where true discipline comes into play. Start by simplifying your life in order to maintain momentum in your own practice. Breathe a bit deeper, declutter your mind, and rid yourself of all that does not serve you. You may notice then that you have more time that you originally thought. I often suggest practicing yoga as soon as you wake up, first thing in the morning. If yoga is a priority in your life, then treat it as such.

Attempt to delay all other distractions, such as checking your phone or e-mail, eating breakfast, or anything that puts the practice secondary. The more we pile on before the practice, the more likely the practice time will just slip away. If you need to wake up an hour earlier to get your yoga done, then set the alarm for that time and go to bed earlier to accommodate. Making time and space for yoga takes it out of the "should" mind-set and places it in the "must" mind-set. In terms of the yoga practice itself, being extremely focused and disciplined does not mean perfecting the most advanced poses. Many times, yoga teachers feel the need to "master" what they consider to be difficult poses. With this mentality, the ego becomes attached to being "more advanced." Identify ego-free goals that you fundamentally believe in. Let your goal be simple: to maintain a daily yoga practice. Remember, the more advanced poses will come, but they should not be the motivation. What matter most are the lessons to be learned along the way, which the practice unfolds for you.

Allow time for meditation. As ajna is a spiritual chakra, it is best balanced through meditation. When we offer students time to focus on the third eye in meditation, students may notice a tingling or pulsating sensation around the area of the forehead. When this happens, it is a sign that this blocked chakra is opening. Here is a simple guided meditation that will create more balance in the third eye and can foster more insight and intuition:

- Sit comfortably in an upright meditative seat.
- Visualize a deep-indigo luminous chakra spinning slowly at the center of your forehead.
- Imagine this indigo light filling your head.
- Now visualize a beam of indigo light shooting down from the midline of the body to the lower five chakras—vishuddha, anahata, manipura, svadhist-hana, and muladhara.
- Now Imagine the light filling your entire body with a radiant energy.
- Meditate like this for five to ten minutes, gradually increasing to twenty minutes.

Tratak Meditation is another meditation practice that will balance the ajna chakra. This meditation promotes intense concentration and also aids in cleansing the eyes, tear ducts, and sinuses.

- Light a candle and place it some three feet away in front of you at eye level.
- Begin meditation by steadily gazing at the flame, trying to blink as sporadically as possible.
- Hold your gaze for approximately two minutes, then gently close your eyes.

- Now see the flame with your mind's eye to strengthen the chakra.
- Open your eyes to gaze at the flame again. This time do it for as long as feels comfortable.
- Close your eyes and see the flame with your mind's eye for as long as you can.
- Progressively increase the amount of time you spend gazing at the candle.

Make your class purposeful. Spontaneity and in-the-moment class sequencing can certainly create a dialogue between teacher and student and have the potential to add value to the practitioner experience. Nonetheless, I am a proponent of the vinyasa krama method of class customization. Vinyasa krama means a step-by-step progression into something or to a certain goal. Vinyasa is the principle of synchronizing movement with the breath, sometimes described as moving in a special and particular way. According to Sri Krishnamacharya, the father of modern yoga, *krama* literally means steps or stages. While karma in general refers to action, krama usually indicates an orderly way of doing a karma or an action. The word *akrama*, the opposite of *krama*, is also used very commonly in India and indicates when something is done in a disorderly, unjust, or unlawful way. To apply vinyasa krama into your sequences means you are planning your classes in an intelligent and methodical way. The flow remains fluid and spontaneous, but the sequence and the substance are never haphazard.

Vinyasa krama is also the art of knowing when you have integrated the proper work of a certain stage of practice or posture and are appropriately ready to move on. I frequently see teachers ignore the importance of this step-by-step integration. For example, leading students into poses like Adho Mukha Vrksasana (handstand) before developing the necessary strength and flexibility in less demanding postures like Adho Mukha Svanasana (downward-facing dog), Sirsasana (headstand), and Bakasana (crane pose), to name a few. This only results in the students struggling, becoming frustrated, or even injuring themselves. When there is strain in a posture, the integration of the previous krama has been ignored. On the other hand, some students may get too comfortable and become stagnant. With proper guidance and awareness of vinyasa krama, this type of student can be given the encouragement to open to a new posture they had written off as beyond their abilities. The high-level organization of vinyasa krama may not be immediately obvious to all the students in the class, but their sixth chakras will experience greater clarity from the mindful movements you offer.

Make eye contact. The old saying that "eyes are a reflection of your inner self" still holds true. Our eyes also reflect our sincerity, integrity, and comfort when communicating with others, which is why having good eye contact while teaching is an indication of strong communication. Traditionally, the yoga student-teacher dynamic was a very sacred relationship. In a one-on-one teaching method of guru to student, you can imagine that plenty of deep connection and eye contact happened. Now that most teachers teach group classes, a lot of the traditional intimacy of student and teacher has been lost, yet when you make eye contact with a person, you are giving him or her your complete attention. You are letting him or her know, without words, that he or she matters. Recall if you have ever had a conversation with someone and noticed that he or she avoided or rarely looked you in the eye. Can you recall the feeling that arose from that type of conversation? Perhaps you thought the person wasn't interested in talking to you, or maybe the person just wasn't friendly. As teachers, we need to consider the classes we teach as a conversation we are having with every single person who shows up. Every student deserves your attention, and lack of eye contact can be interpreted as the teacher being distant, bored, not confident, distracted, or even not friendly. Sure, it can be an overwhelming feeling at times to lock eyes with someone you don't really know, but keep in mind that you have been called to teach yoga, and this requires you to peel away the feelings of shyness and put yourself out there fully. I cannot reiterate enough that the key to truly connecting to another human being is through eye contact. The key to being a highly effective yoga teacher is connecting to your students, and the sensory experience associated with manipura chakra is sight—so look your students in the eyes. As I mentioned before, even just a glance gives them a sense that you care about them.

Let the students go within themselves. Every time I teach, I consider how I can help students go inward. Any student who even slightly touches his or her true self will see a dramatic, positive life change. I have seen so many students' lives change so completely that the teachings of yoga continuously inspire me to make each and every class as badass as I can. The pauses between asanas are an especially important aspect of the overall practice. Always consider that the asanas, even the more challenging ones, are all about bringing students more inward. Allowing them the opportunity to feel the energy of their perfect inward space will help them experience more peace, calmness, and joy, and that will correspond to a greater feeling of awakening and divinity. A certain amount of stillness, according to each student's ability, is required in and after each asana, so the body will gradually take a back seat to the awareness of the inward-flowing and upward-rising energy. You may notice that newer students will have a more difficult time with stillness. This is only natural, as they likely will have limited endurance in the poses and lack of experience in handling stillness and going inward. Do not lose patience with newer yogis who appear restless during moments of stillness. They will eventually learn to turn their minds inward, but only if you offer them a safe and welcoming space to explore the practice. More experienced yogis can handle stillness and may even want more stillness in their practice. An important tool to learning to quiet the mind is to quiet the body; only when the body is quiet can the mind follow. That is why it is so important to offer opportunities to go within, even in the asanas.

Vijnanamaya kosha, the fourth sheath, becomes more relevant with the opportunity to go within, as it is considered the wisdom sheath. Vijnanamaya encompasses intuition and intellect and can be thought of as the aspect of our consciousness that is not entangled in what we are doing or thinking, but rather, is acutely *aware* of what we are doing and thinking. When you've reached the point in your yoga practice where you are much less distracted by random thoughts or occurrences and much less caught up in the anticipation of the next pose, you find you are more able to *feel* the pose. This is the layer where practitioners can gain deeper insights into themselves and the world around them. The spirit of the pose begins to emerge, and the inner voice of "that feels good" becomes louder and louder.

See your students. I know it seems obvious, but what type of investment are you *really* making in your students? Knowing your students is more than knowing their names; it's learning to read both their body language and body mechanics. An important aspect of teacher training is to train the eye of a teacher to detailed observation. When you start to apply this type of approach to your students, you'll notice that Steve is always adding a core sequence before class starts, Dafna is always rubbing her low back on a therapy ball when you offer a resting opportunity, and Diana wears glasses but takes them off when class starts. This type of observation is highly important, like a hidden inventory of little things you are noticing about the students that they aren't even aware of you tuning in to. When we have this global awareness of what is happening with the students, we are better able to give them what they need without having to ask them directly. We may be mindful to add a core engagement for Steve, give a few extra cues in upward-facing dog to ease Dafna's back, or demonstrate closer to Diana to ensure she can see clearly what's going on.

Make sure there is enough time for Savasana. When ajna is in excess, the mind has a tendency to be very busy, rushing from one thought to the next. This feeling of mind chatter can show up for many students during class, and as we discussed from the yoga sutras, the goal of yoga is to cease those mind fluctuations. Leave ample time for rest, and let your students know there is no urgency when in savasana. I would say to spend at least five minutes and up to ten in savasana in a seventy-five-minute class. As I mentioned earlier, yoga is a ritual. It is meant to start with a warm-up, followed by the practice itself, and end with a sort of integration phase for the effects of the postures to seep into the mind and body. Savasana helps achieve that. After a practice that involves stretching, twisting, contracting, and inverting of muscles, savasana allows your body to rest and regroup. It is a perfect end to a satisfying practice. Savasana is often referred to as the most important pose of all, because of its numerous benefits. Here are a few:

- **Brings the body to a meditative state**: The body relaxes and goes into a deep meditative state, which helps repair cells and tissues and releases stress. Savasana allows ultimate relaxation of your body and mind, which is just as essential as exercise and a balanced diet are.

- **Relaxes and calms the body**: Savasana replenishes and rejuvenates the body. Yoga bestows the nervous system with an immense amount of neuromuscular information. Savasana helps your nervous system integrate this information before your mind gets busy with the typical stressors of life. It is a great end to a practice, especially if it has been an intense one. Savasana also gives space and time for the practice to sink in and assimilate into the body. It is a perfect buffer between practice and your daily life.

- **Reduces blood pressure and anxiety**: When your body relaxes and calms down, your blood pressure also slows and relaxes your heart. As a result, students may notice feelings of anxiety abate and are under greater control.

- **Increases energy level**: Savasana is the fastest and safest way to gain instant energy. This few-minute break gives your body an energy boost, thereby increasing your productivity. Some yogis suggest that just a five-minute savasana is the equivalent of two to three hours of deep sleep.

Everyone comes to the mat for their own particular reasons, and the reasons are vast. For some, it is because the asanas give them strength and balance. Some simply find enjoyment in the yoga practice. For others, the journey through yoga is more of a spiritual practice, bringing the union of body, mind, and spirit off the mat and into everyday life. Whatever a student's reasons are for practicing, we need not judge them. Regardless of our own personal reasons, savasana is important, because it allows the students to reap the benefits of the physicality of the poses, but it also enables them to bring yoga from asana into self-awareness. Savasana informs what the students will take from the practice on any given day. If you find yourself with a choice between one more pose or a longer savasana, the latter will always be a better choice.

The Demon of Doubt

As a yoga teacher, you likely will encounter a time when you experience self-doubt and ignore the intuitive wisdom of the sixth chakra. The reality is, not everyone is going to dig your teaching style. Some students you will teach once, and they will never show up again. Some will even walk out of your class early. Don't be discouraged, as none of this is a reason for self-doubt. In the early days of my teaching, I thought that if students never came back, it was a reflection on me. I had to remind myself of the many teachers whose classes *I* only attended once, for a variety of different reasons—though, admittedly, sometimes it was because I didn't connect with their teaching style. This is just evidence that we won't all love the same teacher. Not all students will like you, but that doesn't make you a bad teacher. As a teacher, you will have a unique way of sharing your knowledge that will perfectly fit the way some students want to receive the wisdom. You're meant to serve them, and you're probably not meant to serve those who don't come back to your class. Keep this in mind when fear and doubt try to creep in. As long as you're teaching with love, compassion, and the right knowledge, there's no need for self-doubt. The students who will really benefit from your class will keep coming back. Similar to the strategy discussed to rid yourself of fears, when you witness a seed of doubt being planted, the best approach is to uncover it and bring it to the surface. Write it down or speak your doubts out loud to remove them from your internal awareness. Let them dissolve from your thoughts and patterns.

Reflection:
What is your self-doubt teaching you?

Before You Teach...
One highly effective method for soothing the sixth chakra is to rub the hands together as quickly as possible to generate heat, then place the hands over the eyes. This allows you to experience the leftover vibration created from the friction. This can be done either seated or lying down and will help rid the mind of distracting thoughts. You can also try repeating a sixth-chakra affirmation, such as these:

- "I envision and create beauty and goodness."
- "My imagination is vivid and powerful."
- "I am open to the wisdom within me."
- "I am open to greater spiritual awareness."

Poses for a Sixth-Chakra Sequence

1. Garudasana (eagle pose)
2. Parsvottanasana (intense side-stretch pose)
3. Makarasana (dolphin pose)
4. Pincha Mayurasana (feathered peacock pose)

Seven

FIND YOUR BLISS AND LOVE YOUR YOGA

Wisdom begins at the end.

—DANIEL WEBSTER

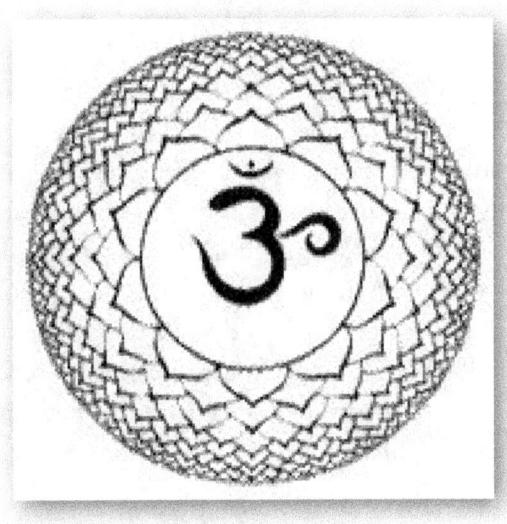

Chakra Seven Overview

Name: Sahasrara (thousandfold)

Element: Thought

Color: Violet or white

Purpose: To understand

Basic Rights: To know and to learn

Properties: Presence, emptiness, understanding, grace, knowledge, awareness

Signs of Deficiency: A closed mind, learning difficulties, rigid belief systems

Signs of Excess: Confusion, excessive attachments, spiritual addiction, prone to over analyzing a situation

Signs of Balance: Wisdom, spiritual connection, open-mindedness, ability to analyze

Demon: Attachment

The seventh chakra, Sahasrara, is referred to as the thousand-petal lotus chakra and is located at the crown of the head. The thousand-petal lotus represents our potential to emerge from the muddy waters of material attachment to find absolute freedom and clarity. The crown chakra rises above the head and connects the physical earth body to the spiritual energetic body. It is said to be our source of enlightenment and spiritual connection to our higher selves and to every being and energy of the universe. Whether you ever reach a true enlightened state in this lifetime is irrelevant. As long as you can just accept that every yoga class you take helps you feel better on a multitude of levels, then that is surely good enough.

When deficient, the sahasrara may cause learning difficulties and can trap energy in the lower chakras. In excess, the seventh chakra has a tendency to pull us out of the earthbound experience, leading to inaction or inability to follow through with material tasks. Similarly, overintellectualization is a symptom of too much energy circulating in the crown and can produce a racing mind, insomnia, or even nightmares. Balance in sahasrara is the realization that you are pure consciousness, undivided and all expansive. It is often described as being like a drop in the ocean; you are a part of that ocean that contains and encompasses every aspect of consciousness.

The seventh chakra opens the gateway of directing our attention and allows us to become the masters of our consciousness. Learning to control your attention is a goal, but it's also a result of a consistent yoga practice. Patanjali's Yoga Sutras outline the eight limbs of yoga, which essentially give a detailed outline of the yogic path that leads to the awakening of the seventh chakra. There are many books on yoga philosophy that can discuss the eight limbs in great detail; however, I will touch on these limbs briefly, as they form the structure of upper-chakra awareness and practice.

Patanjali's Eight-Limbed Path of Yoga

Yama	Universal morality
Niyama	Personal observances
Asanas	Physical postures
Pranayama	Breathing practices
Pratyahara	Withdrawal of the senses
Dharana	Concentration
Dhyana	Meditation
Samadhi	Union with the divine

The first limb, yama, usually refers to vows, disciplines, or practices that are primarily concerned with how we interact with the world around us. There are five yamas, including Ahimsa (nonharming), Satya (truthfulness), Asteya (nonstealing), Brahmacharya (moderation or correct use of energy), and Aparigraha (nongreed or nonhoarding). These principles lay the foundation so we can be yogi off the mat in our daily interactions. In B. K. S. Iyengar's translation of the sutras, *Light On Yoga,* he explains that Yamas are "unconditioned by time, class, and place," meaning that no matter who we are, where we come from, or how many times a week we practice yoga, we can all still strive to live a life with yama as the basis of our choices and interactions. Therefore, the premise of practicing yama is if we can learn to be compassionate and honest, while using our energy in a worthwhile way, we will not only be benefiting ourselves but also everyone and everything around us.

Yamas: Ethical Rules

- Ahimsa (nonharming) is usually translated as *nonviolence*, but this idea goes far and beyond the limited thought of not killing others, particularly in the role of a yoga teacher. Extending this compassion to all living creatures is dependent on our understanding and acknowledgment of the underlying union of all beings, with the scope of understanding way beyond our friends, family, and pets. When we begin to recognize that the rivers of the earth are no different from the blood flowing through our own veins, it becomes very natural to extend compassion without any sense of doubt or restraint. Coinciding with the realization of oneness, it becomes increasingly difficult to remain indifferent to the problems and injustices of the world. In considering ahimsa as a yoga teacher, it's helpful to ask yourself if your thoughts and actions are fostering the growth and well-being of all things.
- Satya (truthfulness) urges us to live and speak our truth at all times. Walking the path of truth is a hard one, especially while respecting Patanjali's first yama, ahimsa. Since ahimsa must be practiced first, we must be careful to not speak a truth if we know it will cause

harm to another. Living in your truth not only creates respect, honor, and integrity but also provides the vision to clearly see the higher truths of the yogic path.

- Asteya (nonstealing) is best defined as not taking what is not freely given. While this may on the surface seem easy to accomplish, when we look further, this yama can be quite challenging to practice. On a personal level, the practice of asteya entails not committing theft physically and not causing or approving of anyone else doing so in thought, word, or deed. While not easy, practicing asteya encourages generosity and overcomes greed. As Patanjali teaches us, "When asteya is firmly established in a yogi, all jewels will become present to him/her" (Yoga Sutra 2.37).

- Brahmacharya (moderation) states that when we have control over our physical impulses of excess, we attain knowledge, vigor, and increased energy. To break the bonds that attach us to our excesses and addictions, we need both courage and will. Every time we overcome impulses of excessive sensory fulfillment, we become stronger, healthier, and wiser. One of the main goals in yoga is to create and maintain balance. And the simplest method for achieving balance is by practicing brahmacharya, creating moderation in all our activities.

- Aparigraha (nonhoarding) urges us to let go of everything we do not need, possessing only as much as is necessary. Yogic scripture teaches us that worldly objects cannot be possessed at all, as they are all subject to change and ultimately will be destroyed. When we become greedy and covetous, we lose the ability to see our one eternal possession, the true self. Essentially, when we cling to what we have, we lose the ability to be open to receive what we actually need.

Niyama, the second limb of Patanjali's eight-limbed path usually refers to duties directed toward ourselves. The prefix "ni" is a Sanskrit verb that means "inward" or "within" and is traditionally practiced by those who wish to build strong moral character. Interestingly, the niyamas closely relate to the koshas, our sheaths or layers leading from the physical body to the essence within. As you'll notice, when we work with the niyamas, from saucha to isvara pranidhana, we are guided from the grossest aspects of ourselves to the deepest truths within. There are five niyamas, including saucha (cleanliness), santosha (contentment), tapas (discipline or fire), svadhyaya (self-study and study of spiritual texts), and isvara pranidhana (devotion and surrender to a higher power).

Niyamas: Observances

- Saucha (cleanliness) is a central aim of many yogic techniques and is the first principle of Patanjali's five niyamas. The yogis discovered that impurities in both our external environment and our internal body adversely affect our state of mind and prevent the attainment of real wisdom and spiritual liberation.

The practices of asana, pranayama, and meditation cleanse and purify the body and mind and strengthen their capacity to maintain a pure state of being. We must also consciously work at surrounding ourselves with a pure environment (including food, drink, friends, entertainment, and habits) to not add any external impurities back into our bodies or minds.

- Santosha (contentment) is not craving what we do not have as well as not coveting the possessions of others. Yoga teaches us that when we are perfectly content with all that life gives us, we attain true joy and happiness. It is easy for the mind to become fooled into thinking we can attain lasting happiness through the possession of objects and material goods, but both our personal experience and the teachings of the sages prove that the happiness gained through materialism is only temporary. Practicing contentment frees us from the unnecessary suffering of always wanting things to be different and instead fills us with gratitude and joy for all life's blessings.

- Tapas (discipline) is a yogic practice of intense self-discipline and attainment of willpower. Basically, tapas is doing something you do not want to do but know will have a positive effect on your life. When our willpower conflicts with the desire of our mind, an internal "fire" is created, which illuminates and burns up our mental and physical impurities. The yogis say that tapas transforms and purifies us, while controlling our unconscious impulses and poor behavior patterns. Tapas is what builds the dedication and personal strength that allows us to become dedicated to our yoga practice.

- Svadhyaya (self-study) is the ability to see our true divine nature through the contemplation of our life's lessons, as exemplified through the truths revealed in spiritual texts. Life presents an endless opportunity to learn about ourselves, and our flaws and mistakes give us the opportunity to grow and learn. When we examine our actions, they become like a mirror that reveals our conscious and unconscious motives, thoughts, and desires more clearly.

- Ishvara Pranidhana (devotion) is the dedication, devotion, and surrender of the fruits of one's practice to a higher power. Patanjali teaches us that to reach the goal of yoga, we must dissolve our egocentric nature and let go of our constant identification with who we think we are. Our yoga practice should be seen as an offering to something greater than ourselves. Through this simple act of dedication, we become reminded of our connection to our higher power, and our yoga practice becomes sacred and filled with inner peace, deeper consciousness, and love.

The foundational limbs of Patanjali's eightfold path of yoga, yama and niyama, create a solid foundation and strong container for the yogi to move into the deeper stages of yoga with focus, inner strength, and success. Practicing the yamas and niyamas is a process. If taking on yama and niyama as part of a practice seems daunting, take it slowly. Work with one yama or niyama at a time and proceed with compassion and without attachment to perfection. As Swami Sri Kripalvanandji said, "When you pick one petal from the garland of yamas and niyamas, the entire garland will follow."

Asana, or the physical aspect of yoga, is the third step on the path to yogic freedom. The translation of asana isn't handstand, full split, or crow pose. Interesting enough, it actually means "seat," so the physical asana practice is really just a preparation for being able to sit in meditation. Once the practitioner realizes this, he or she can easily let go of attachments to fancy poses that really don't get us any closer to enlightenment. The only alignment instruction Patanjali gives for asana is "sthira sukham asanam," meaning the posture should be steady and comfortable. While traditional texts such as the Hatha Yoga Pradipika list many postures, such as Padmasana (lotus pose) and Virasana (hero pose), suitable for meditation, this text also tells us that the most important posture is in fact sthira sukhasana—a posture the practitioner can hold comfortably and motionlessly. You may ask yourself or your students to tune in to how many poses they can sustain while truly being comfortable and steady.

The next limb, pranayama (as we mentioned earlier), refers to breathing practices and control of the breath. The physical act of working with different breathing techniques can alter the mind in a myriad of ways. There are practices designed to calm the mind, as well as more stimulating techniques. Our breathing patterns can change our state of being, but it's up to us whether we perceive this as controlling the way we feel or as freeing us from the habits of the mind.

Pratya means to withdraw or draw in, and the second part *ahara* refers to anything we "take in" by ourselves, such as the various aspects of our five senses. The practice of drawing inward may include focusing on the way we're breathing, so this limb would relate directly to the practice of pranayama as well. The practice of pratyahara changes our state of mind so that we become so absorbed in what it is we're focusing on that things outside of ourselves no longer bother us. This also increases our capacity for meditation and eliminating distracting thoughts.

The last three limbs are most highly intertwined with the upper chakras, as attention is being brought to the true aspect of yoga, which is union. The next limb, Dharana, means "focused concentration." *Dha* means "holding or maintaining," and *rana* means "something else." Closely linked to the previous two limbs, dharana and pratyahara are essential parts of the same aspect. In order to focus on something, the senses must withdraw so that all attention is put into the focal point of concentration. In order to have the ability to draw the senses in, we must focus and concentrate intensely and with intention.

The seventh limb is Dhyana or "meditative absorption," as in this limb, we become consumed by the focus of our meditation. Focused attention is necessary before one can experience meditation. In meditation, we become aware of the infinite nature of consciousness, and the feeling of *I-ness* or separation dissolves.

This leads us to samadhi, which is often translated as "bliss" or "enlightenment." This is the final step of the journey of Patanjali's Yoga Sutras, yet it doesn't refer to floating away in a state of ecstasy—sorry! In dissecting that word, we see that this final limb is made up of two words: *sama* meaning "equal or same" and *dhi* meaning "to see." This idea of bliss is often called *realization*, because reaching Samadhi is not about reaching ultimate joy or ecstasy; rather, it's about realizing the beauty in the life that lies in front of you. It is about a release of the disturbances of the mind, without our experiences being conditioned by likes, dislikes, or habits and without the need to judge or become attached to any particular aspect of life. Now *that* is bliss.

Seventh Chakra Yoga-Teaching Tips

Live your dharma. The word *dharma*, like so many Sanskrit terms, has different meanings depending on context and who's defining it. Dharma is often defined as "duty"; however, it is much more than this. *Dharma* comes from the root "dhri," which means to uphold or uplift, and dharma literally refers to "that which upholds righteousness." A sense of righteousness and of purpose and inspiration is extremely significant on the spiritual path of teaching yoga. Dharma can mean "law of the universe" and/or one's own individual purpose or mission. Dharma might be considered to have two distinct, yet mutually supportive components: (1) our personal or individual dharma (svadharma) of unique qualities (e.g., talents, gifts, traits, and abilities) that help to define our life's path and (2) our Sat Dharma or "true" dharma, that path of self-realization that is everyone's birthright and shared by all beings. When your life's purpose is connected to your svadharma and sat dharma, it brings you joy and fulfillment. When you are disconnected from dharma, your purpose may feel confused, and your efforts to be your happiest may feel difficult or even prevented.

> *It is better to do your own*
> *dharma even imperfectly,*
> *than someone else's dharma perfectly.*

—BHAGAVAD GITA

The idea of "living your dharma" has historically meant that a person lives in a way that is in accordance with the laws of destiny. In India, this was traditionally interpreted to mean living according to your caste, gender, or some other constricting factor. But another, perhaps truer, interpretation of dharma is the idea of simply doing what you were meant to do. Living your dharma means living your true purpose and expressing it in the world, while truly believing there is nothing else you would rather be doing with your life.

Remember what inspired you to teach in the first place, meditate on it, write it down, and refer to it often. Teaching a great yoga class takes every bit of energy, focus, and intuitive insight we can muster. Become very clear about your teaching vision, and use this as a filter for making decisions and taking action. Let teaching yoga be but a single part of your living purpose, or dharma, where passion, professionalism, and blessedness to serve all intersect.

Avoid teacher burnout. Burnout in teachers is particularly problematic, because in order to do your job effectively, you need to be fully present. You need to be open and prepared. We don't have the liberty of spending our days daydreaming or hiding in a cubicle. Teacher burnout usually happens when a teacher becomes so overzealous with the thought of teaching that they pack in too many classes, reducing the quality of each offering. When you start to leave at the last possible minute to teach a class, can't stand the sequence you are teaching, find yourself refraining from talking to your students, or haven't had a day off in months, it's very likely that you have been experiencing yoga-teacher burnout. Be aware of the warning signs, such as feeling uninspired, having difficulty sleeping, waking up tired, and no longer prioritizing your personal practice. Yoga-teacher burnout is a real syndrome and one that can lead you to question if you're rightly fulfilling your dharma; however, if you're alert to the early signs of burnout, you can water the flames when they show up.

Teaching yoga can be isolating. Yoga teachers can be on the run so much, and aside from passing interactions before and after class, it may be hard to find the time to have a meaningful conversation. Set up a time to meet with someone you like and admire, maybe your mentor, and be honest about how you feel. Be open to whatever feedback you may receive. Try to attend a workshop or training that can ignite the spark in your teaching. In this day and age, it is possible to learn from renowned teachers through a variety of online resources available right in the comfort of your own home. It can be a very energizing feeling to have a new sequence or focus to bring to your classes, so utilize the resources that are readily available.

Use at least one day per week to do something just for yourself. This could be a walk in the park, a chat with a friend in a coffee shop, a massage, or a morning to sleep in. Perhaps most importantly, be honest with yourself and take time to explore the root cause of your burnout. Teaching yoga full-time can be a rewarding yet challenging path from a financial and emotional standpoint. You may spend a lot of time traveling around from studio to studio, and being in a position of support to others can be draining on your own needs. You also need to stay open to learning and need to find the balance of your own practice while dealing with any financial implications this teaching path may incur. All these factors can contribute to burnout and stress. Stay open to other ways of expressing your passion. If you find that you're constantly feeling exhausted, maybe it's time to think of a new way to integrate teaching yoga into your life. Consider moving to a full-time job while teaching an evening class or two as a temporary shift or option if you feel a strong desire to create more overall balance in your life.

Live your yoga off the mat. It's easy to find a sense of tranquility in a yoga studio, surrounded by peaceful decor and the soothing sounds that help to guide you into relaxation. But what happens after you teach? Do you take what you have taught in class and apply it to your life off the mat, or do you fall right back into your old habits, like getting pissed off in traffic jams, feeling frazzled about work stuff, or being nitpicky with your partner?

As yoga teachers, we have the opportunity every time we teach to learn something new about ourselves and the way we move, think, act, and breathe. We can have some incredible "a-ha" moments during class, but the real benefits come when we can take those moments with us outside of the studio. Breathing is the most important aspect of life, but how often are you really partaking in conscious full breaths outside of teaching or taking yoga classes? Become curious about how you breathe in the same way you offer when you teach. Tune in to your breath several times a day. Notice the quality of its natural flow, and see how it changes at different times. The quality and flow of your breath will most often reflect how you are feeling internally, so if you need to, use that awareness to deepen and steady your breath to feel calmer and more centered.

You don't have to be in a yoga pose to notice the position of your body and how you naturally stand and move. Take with you the way you teach your students to be more aware of their alignment during an asana. Use that same sense of awareness as you move throughout your day. You may be quite surprised at some of your habitual ways of moving your body. Next time you're waiting in line at Starbucks, instead of pulling out your iPhone to check your e-mail, why not tune in and notice what's going on with the position of your body? If you favor one side as you stand, make adjustments and come back to a place of balance. If you hold unnecessary tension in your jaw, shoulders, or hands, then use the breath to soften and let go. Yoga is so much more than what happens on the mat; if we let it, it can enhance the way we interact with the world. As Baron Baptiste says, go from *doing* yoga to *being* yoga!

The final kosha, anandamaya kosha, offers the feeling of wholeness and bliss. It creates the sense of arriving at your destination, even if only for a moment. Anandamaya can be experienced when you are wholly immersed in what you're doing—when you no longer separate yourself from your experiences. Be aware of the moments that act as opportunities to live in this wholeness and the joy the practice can create for you.

Evolve as a teacher. In a world with more and more yoga teachers, you must be clear on your message as a teacher. Think of what is important to you, then continue to evolve and advance in your craft. In advancing your teachings, you will go deeper into the practice and begin to teach with more clarity and vision. This deepening of your understanding will give you more confidence, greater stability, and a foundation from which to make more intuitive decisions. Study with those who have wisdom of experience that is more expansive than your own, and take full advantage of their experience. Yoga is believed to be over five thousand years old, so there is a lot to learn. You may feel you are drawn to energy and would like to dive deeper into that subtle aspect of yoga, perhaps by exploring chakra theories and reiki. Maybe your goal is to become more knowledgeable in ways to alleviate physical pain and suffering. You can expand in working with the human body and physical anatomy, learn how to work with injuries, and most importantly discover how to prevent them. You could also pursue teaching yoga more therapeutically, finding a niche concept or population you would like to work with. Nowadays, there is yoga for kids, yoga for pregnant women, couples yoga, yoga for trauma, yoga for anxiety, chair yoga, water yoga, yoga for dogs—you name it, and there is yoga for it. Whatever you decide as an area you would like to evolve in, remember to constantly show up at your best, leave your drama at home, and strive to get better at serving your students.

Perhaps your own evolution in yoga can mean venturing into an alternate path or incorporating other paths of yoga into your practice. Having a physical asana practice constitutes Hatha yoga; however, there are other main paths that can be beneficial in deepening your knowledge and understandings beyond just the physical.

Bhakti is the yoga of devotion, ultimately to the divine. In today's vibrant world, with all its confusion and chaos, many people believe Bhakti is the easiest of the paths to follow. It can be practiced by anyone—regardless of mental or physical abilities—and doesn't involve extensive yogic practices. Bhakti is the path of love, which removes jealousy, hatred, lust, anger, egoism, pride, and arrogance. It replaces those feelings with feelings of joy, divine ecstasy, bliss, peace, and wisdom. The spiritual texts tell us bhakti is already within us; it's just been lying dormant in our hearts since the beginning of creation. This feeling of love and devotion is often hidden by layers of ignorance and suffering; however, no matter what you do or where you go, this thread of divine connection can never be broken.

Bhakti teaches that to be *in* love with someone or something creates separation; instead, Bhakti is to *be* love—to be intoxicated with it. It is the idea of being in love with love itself. Practices of a bhakti yogi include songs and chants sung in praise of the divine, often in a kirtan or call-and-response fashion. The bhakti finds surrender by being open to everything, striving to be pure in thoughts, words, and actions.

Karma yoga is another path that the Bhagavad Gita discusses in-depth. *Karma* means "action," and Karma yoga is performing action without attachment to the outcome. It is the path of selfless service or Seva. In Karma yoga, you cease to identify with the ego, and all action is seen as an offering to the divine. The practitioner strives to be purified of egoism, hatred, jealousy, selfishness, and similar negative qualities so space can be created for humility, pure love, sympathy, tolerance, and compassion. Karma yoga is "doing the right thing." It means following one's dharma (true purpose) and accepting whatever comes, without expectation of payment, thanks, or recognition. A karma yogi lives his life with great passion but is dispassionate about the outcome. He rejoices in others' successes and speaks as truthfully as possible.

Jnana yoga is the path of knowledge or wisdom. It is the means to enlightenment through the process of reason—particularly the process of discrimination between what is real and not real and what is true and untrue through study of the spiritual texts and self-inquiry. Jnana yoga is said to be the most difficult path, because it uses the mind and intellect to finally realize we are one with the divine. The Upanishads call it the "razor's edge," where the ego is always trying to knock us off. It requires great strength of character, willpower, and intellect. The Jnana yogi studies the words of the great masters and spiritual texts in his or her traditions and seeks to find answers without judgment.

Raja yoga means the "Royal Path." Just as a king maintains control over his kingdom, you must maintain control over your own "kingdom"—the vast territory of your mind and your thoughts. Raja yoga is the path of meditation, mantras, and techniques described in Patanjali's Yoga Sutras. The premise in Raja yoga is to keep the body and mind still and pure, so the true self can shine forth. Raja yoga is the path most favored by Westerners, because it can be practiced by almost everyone, requiring no belief or particular faith. The Raja yogi keeps harmony with nature's rhythms and takes responsibility for his or her choices and life outcomes. He or she avoids distractions by training the mind through meditation.

Kundalini yoga is a blend of Bhakti yoga, Raja yoga, and Shakti yoga (the expression of power and energy). The purpose of kundalini yoga is to provide a modality by which people can free themselves from karma (the lasting effects of past actions) and realize their life purpose. The term *kundalini* means a spiritual energy or life force located at the base of the spine, which is usually conceptualized as a coiled serpent. The practice of kundalini yoga is supposed to arouse the sleeping kundalini serpent from its coiled base through the six chakras that reside along the spine and through the seventh chakra, or crown. Many of the physical postures in kundalini yoga are designed to activate the navel, spine, and focal points on meridians (energy points). Through pranayama and the application of yogic locks of energy (bandhas), the release, direction, and control of the flow of kundalini energy is achieved.

The Demon of Attachment

One common symptom of both deficient and excessive energy in the seventh chakra is susceptibility to attachment. As you may have discovered already, when you try to hold on too tightly to anything—whether to relationships or to material items—the grasping often leads only to the demolition of those very things we most covet. When sahasrara is blocked or congested, energy remains trapped in the lower chakras, where attachments such as greed and excessive desire may result. If we are excessive in the crown chakra, there can be a tendency to overidentify with our present reality, which can leave us stagnant and unable to move forward. As a yoga teacher, this may show up as becoming too concerned with your teacher identity or determining your self-worth based on how busy your classes are or aren't. In the Bhagavad Gita, Krishna shares perhaps one of the most important teachings of all: "A gift is pure when it is given from the heart to the right person at the right time and at the right place, and when we expect nothing in return." What Krishna is essentially saying is that we should never concern ourselves with the outcome of a situation or action; we should concern ourselves only with what we are doing, and more specifically, with the intention behind it. Let go of worrying about recognition of your actions, stop wondering if you are "good enough," and trust that you have been called to share your gifts by something far grander than yourself. This is how you can pursue your dharma or duty of teaching yoga, as it aligns with aparigraha or nonattachment. Have faith that you have been called to teach and have a gift to share. Otherwise, why would you be teaching?

Reflection:

Examine your attachments to people, places, money, being right, freedom, suffering, success, children, the past, and the future. If some attachments are particularly strong, write about them at length. Consider ways you can relinquish them.

Before You Teach...

Get upside down! By positioning the heart above the head, you supply a greater flow of blood to the heart, and this increase in blood volume signals a slowing of the heartbeat and activates the parasympathetic (peaceful) nervous system. Therefore, inversions prepare the body for meditation, allowing the body to drop into stillness more easily. Enjoy a brief inverted posture before you teach to shift your energetic awareness in preparation for leading the class into their moving meditation. On your busy days, conserve some vital energy by practicing a more cooling or restorative inversion, such as legs up a wall or viparita karani, with a block under the sacrum. In *Eastern Body, Western Mind*, Anodea Judith explains, "Restoration of the seventh chakra is about awakening to the reality of our spiritual nature. We open this chakra by developing the capacity for stillness, for which there is no better tool than meditation." Therein lies the answer to balancing chakra seven: meditate daily.

Poses for a Seventh-Chakra Sequence

1. Sirsasana (headstand)
2. Seated meditation
3. Viparita Karani (block under the sacrum with legs elevated or legs up a wall)
4. Padmasana (lotus pose)
5. Baddha Konasana (bound-angle pose)

Eight

Chakra Meditation

To close out the thoughts and discussions offered in this book, please use this guided chakra meditation as an additional tool for yourself and students. I look forward to continued discussions about the yoga teaching profession and business of yoga as it aligns with the spiritual yogic texts and philosophies. (((OM)))

Allow your eyes to comfortably close, and come down into your breath, into your body, relax your belly, soften your mind.

Feel supported and connected to the ground beneath you. Let it take on the totality of your weight.

Bring awareness to the sounds around you - let them be there.

Notice the air touching the surface of your body.

Imagine the sky above, and the horizons stretching all the way round you. Feel the supportive nature of everything around you.

Let your mind empty all that it no longer needs; let those thoughts flow out of you. Release from your body what it no longer needs, let it go.

Let go of your day, where you have been, what you did, and instead, bring your intention to your center. Ground yourself in this moment, right here, right now.

Become aware of the rise and fall of your breath, the way it comes and goes, the sensation of it, it's sound and temperature.

Breathe down to where the weight of your body rests, below the base of your spine – to your root. Breathe into your base. Let it soften and gently expand with your breath, take in all its nourishment and life force energy.

Invite in the color red – the color of the earth. Imagine covering your root with red: a color of empowerment, embodiment, and grounding. Silently say the words: "I am here, I have a right to be here, just as I am. The earth supports me."

When you are ready, allow your awareness to move up to your belly, just below your navel – to your chakra of emotional intelligence, choice, creativity, movement and pleasure.

Breathe into your chakra of sweetness, let it gently soften and expand on your breath, take in it's nourishment and life force energy. Invite in orange – the color of the setting sun. Let your second chakra be fed by saying the words: "I honor my needs. I allow myself to be nourished and fulfilled."

When you are ready move your awareness up to the soft area below your breastbone, to your Solar Plexus - your chakra of personal strength and power.

Breathe into this place. Allow your solar plexus to soften and expand with your breath. Invite in the color yellow — the color of sunshine. Let your third chakra take what it needs, as you say the words, "I am enough, I am more than enough."

When you are ready bring your awareness up to the center of your chest- to your Heart- your chakra of compassion and unconditional love.

Gently breathe into your heart. Let it soften and expand with your breath. Invite in green - the color of nature and spring. Bathe your heart center with nourishment, renewal, and healing. Say the words "I am loved. I allow myself to give and receive love freely."

Take your time, but move up to your neck — to your Throat - your chakra of self-expression and personal will.

Allow your throat center to soften, expand and b-r-e-a-t-h-e. Invite in blue — the color of sky. Breathe into your throat elements of opening, and freedom of self-expression and creativity. Say the words "I hear and speak my truth. I express myself freely. I allow myself to go with the flow of life."

When you are ready, take your focus up to your forehead - between your eyebrows - to your third eye — your chakra of wisdom and intuition, gently allowing it to soften and expand.

Invite in the color indigo - the velvety color of night sky. Imagine elements of balance and clarity being brought into your life. Let your third eye take what it needs. Say the words, "Everything is unfolding as it should."

Moving up, in your own time, to the top of your head- to your crown, your chakra of oneness.

Gently invite in a color of light violet above the crown of your head. Invite harmony and restoration into your life. Say the words "I am one with the Universe."

When you are ready, come back to the ebb and flow of your breath, back to your center. Breathe into your core. Say the words "I am whole. I am perfect just as I am."

Allow the energy of the words to bathe your body, mind, emotions, and spirit. Take what you need.

In your own time become aware of the air on the surface of your body. Notice he sounds around you, near and in the distance.

Become aware again of the support beneath you. Notice how you feel. Hold yourself with loving kindness, for the beautiful and unique being that you are.

When you are ready you can draw this meditation to a close.

Nine

Resources

Stay Connected

Follow and engage with our community on social media:

Facebook: www.facebook.com/danahotyoga
www.facebook.com/dontbeanassholeyogateacher

Instagram: www.instagram.com/dana_hot_yoga/

For more information on how to be the most successful and badass yoga teacher you can be, check out the book *Don't Be an Asshole Yoga Teacher.*

About the Author

Dr. Lisa Dana Mitchell has more than five hundred hours of training and years of professional experience as a teacher and student of yoga.

On top of all her experience and training, for the last ten years, she has co-owned three Philadelphia area yoga studios, where she cofounded and directs the Dana Hot Yoga 200-Hour Teacher Training Program. She also participates in International Yoga Retreats around the world.

Mitchell is the author of *Don't Be an Asshole Yoga Teacher*.